Eat Yourself Well

Simple changes for
better health

D1425196

BERNADETTE BOHAN

Gill & Macmillan

Gill & Macmillan
Hume Avenue
Park West
Dublin 12
www.gillmacmillanbooks.ie

© Bernadette Bohan 2013

978 07171 5639 9

Print origination by Carole Lynch
Printed and bound by TJ International, Cornwall
Indexed by Cliff Murphy

This book is typeset in Adobe Garamond 12pt.

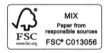

*The paper used in this book comes from the wood
pulp of managed forests. For every tree felled, at least
one tree is planted, thereby renewing natural resources.*

A CIP catalogue record for this book is available
from the British Library.

5 4 3

To my readers, whose love and support means
so much to me.

To Gerard, Richard, Sarah and Julie –
thank you for your love and patience.

To my dear friend Geraldine, you rock.

To Peter for your encouragement.

To Michael Gill, many thanks for making this possible.

Note from the publisher

Information given in this book is not intended to
be taken as a replacement for medical advice.
Any person with a condition requiring medical attention
should consult a qualified medical practitioner or therapist.

Contents

Introduction

'*The future depends on what you do in the present.*'

MAHATMA GANDHI

I have tried! I really have tried to get healthy and lose some weight, BUT nothing's worked! Six days ago, with great enthusiasm and the best of intentions, I decided I was going to change my ways. I was going to make it to the gym, I was going to eat more healthily, and I was definitely going to cut back on sugar and coffee. There was going to be no more feeling sluggish and tired in the afternoon. I hate dieting and keeping track of everything I put in my mouth – and it's so annoying to stand on the weighing scales and feel constantly disappointed. I will get rid of this spare tyre if it's the last thing I do.

I have become so fixated on counting calories, checking the fat and sugar contents of food and trying to figure out:

- What foods have the fewest calories?
- If I cut out dairy, will I get enough calcium?
- Will I get enough proteins if I don't eat meat?

This is what I promised myself six days ago, and – would you believe it – so far, I have achieved nothing. What happened to all those good intentions? Well for one, there was the unforeseen trip to the dentist with Sarah when she woke with a toothache. Then I had to drop Richard to the other side of the city for a football match. I had two parent–teacher meetings, plus all the rest to contend with. Can you blame me? I have been so busy with the kids. It is non-stop, there are just not enough hours in the day. I suppose you could say I am a typical mum, so caught up in the routine of housework, preparing meals and spending time in the car ferrying the kids about that I don't have a lot of time to take care of myself. But really I know I should have done better.

Never mind, all is not lost. I am going to make a fresh start *again* tomorrow.

Does all this sound familiar? Well that was my life some years back, I was finding it impossible to get to grips with changing my eating habits. Then, just as I was trying to get my act together, life dealt me a severe blow – I was diagnosed with cancer for a second time.

If I am truly honest, by saying I was too busy, I was only making excuses for myself. In truth, I was so used to 'normal' food that I really didn't want to know any nutritional details because I knew that if it made sense, I would have to take it on board and make an effort to change my diet.

Looking back now, I wonder if I would have succeeded in turning my life around without that wake-up call, or would I still be dabbling at trying to improve my health? The problem was that I knew a bit about being healthy, but I did not know enough. Apart from the odd health book I had flicked through or the occasional article in a magazine, I had never really made it my business to find out what it takes for the body to function correctly. Although I genuinely thought I was leading a healthy lifestyle, I realise now that I wasn't. It turned out that I was not eating nearly as well as I thought I was. I think if I had understood – and I mean *really* understood – how food affects our health, I might have been more determined to get it right.

When the cancer came back, I had a massive incentive to change my lifestyle – no buts and no excuses. In an effort to become informed, I read tons of books and attended just as many lectures. I found it very confusing when one expert said one thing and then another disagreed. What was I to do? How on earth was I going to get this right? It was a minefield of contradictions and confusion.

I decided to crack on and do the best I could. I set about adding foods to my diet that were more nourishing. I started juicing fruits and vegetables, and I cleaned the water coming into the house. I threw away all the toiletries that contained harmful ingredients and started to take a lot more care of myself, and I mastered one step before I tackled another.

Mind you, despite the confusion, the education I received from the books and seminars was an eye-opener for me. It sparked a true life change and altered my whole perception of health and led me to the healthy lifestyle that I have managed to maintain for the past fourteen years. That education has been one of the key factors that has taught me a common-sense approach to better health. Taking action somehow made me feel more in control. It gave me back control over my life, something that seemed to be stripped away when I was diagnosed with cancer.

Shortly after I began to eat these nourishing foods, I saw real results. My health improved greatly, my painful arthritis disappeared, I gave up wearing my reading glasses and, as an added bonus, my spare tyre melted away – and all of these changes have remained constant over the intervening years. Thankfully, I am now healthier and slimmer without dieting. The beauty and simplicity of this plan is that it is a lifestyle change, and not just a trendy temporary diet that doesn't have lasting results.

I have come to realise that the smallest changes can have the biggest impact. True health must be earned, there are no magic pills or cures that can replace the wonderful foods that nature has given to us.

The moral of my story is start today, not tomorrow. If only I had known how much these simple changes would improve my life, I wouldn't have made so many excuses and would have started much sooner.

I realise that you may know some of the information in this book already, but I want to explain what I have learned in detail so that you fully understand how these simple steps will transform your life for the better. This is not a diet, it's a way of life, and it will help you to improve your food choices, break harmful habits and create better ones.

The process of eating healthily doesn't have to be complicated. In fact, as I have said repeatedly, the secret is to keep it simple – that way you are far more likely to succeed. This book will help you see through the clutter of complicated information that surrounds food. I hope it will become the foundation of your informed decision-making and will help you to take responsibility for your health.

Over the past thirteen years, I have taught thousands of people how to make the simple changes that I will explain in this book. Spreading the word on the benefits of healthy living has become my passion. I want to pass on the common-sense steps that helped me return to good health to give you easy ways to improve your health and wellbeing. I am teaching a sustainable, uncomplicated lifestyle that promotes eating foods in a way that is as close as possible to their natural state – not processed, sprayed or treated with growth hormones and antibiotics or chemicals but the way that Mother Nature intended us to eat them. If, like me, you have made repeated resolutions to get healthy but have lacked the motivation, willpower and knowledge, then this book will get you on track.

Eat Yourself Well has everything you need to achieve real health and shed those extra pounds. There are tips for every area – including juicing, weaning yourself off sugar, dairy and coffee, getting your family on board, losing weight, and eating out – small and attainable tips that *work*. These tips are gathered from my own personal experiences and also from the thousands of readers and students who have shared a lot of practical information about how they have successfully incorporated this programme into their everyday lives. Their experiences have helped shape this road map to better health, which will help you to cultivate a healthy lifestyle in a permanent way, not just for a week or two.

This lifestyle has become second nature to me and I no longer allow life's distractions to interfere with my ability to take care of myself. Yet, I know from my own experience how hard it is to get your head around modifying your eating habits. I have written this book in response to the thousands of questions I have received. It is a hands-on, practical guide that addresses the details and questions that crop up time after time when I am teaching. There is a quick reference section at the end of each chapter to help you remember the information discussed and these guidelines will keep you on track. The book is packed with tips and some of my latest, most favourite recipes. I hope it will give you the direction and guidance you need to improve your health for the better.

Let me share the lessons I have learned along my journey to health, which can be summed up in this simple message: 'When you take an active role in your health, you can make a difference – a huge difference.'

Thank you so much for reading, enjoy and keep well.

Bernadette

1

Getting started

*'Without continual growth and progress, such words as
'improvement', 'achievement' and 'success' have no meaning.'*

BENJAMIN FRANKLIN

The essential ingredient for good health is education. Becoming educated is a crucial step to understanding your health, otherwise health matters will always remain a mystery. How can you make changes to your lifestyle if you don't understand what those changes will mean? Health education provides you with the know-how to influence your life for the better – just as a lack of knowledge can lead you to make the wrong decisions. I am a massive believer in giving people information so that they can make better decisions. It is so important that people take responsibility for their own health and this means that they have to do some research, listen to all sides of an argument and then make informed decisions. When people are told what to do, they will do it for a while, but when they know *why* they are doing something, they make lasting changes.

To avoid reverting to old habits, you first need knowledge and understanding, and then the tools to make changes and create habits that will give you the energy you need and the health you desire. Obtaining this essential information will help you to decide what is right for you.

Invest a bit of time to becoming clued up on your health. I am not asking you to accept my word blindly – I know how important it is to find something you trust. So use your instincts and, above all, take action and stick with it. When you understand how it all works, you will see the sense in adjusting the way you live. It makes perfect sense to hold on to your most valuable asset – your health.

My advice is to become interested in your health before you have to. Make your biggest investment in the one place you must live for the rest of your life – your body. I promise it will be the best investment you will ever make. If you want to buy a car you will save money, take out a loan, check out the internet and go from garage to garage to test drive the car you want. You invest time and energy in that new car. The same should apply to your health. Your level of success will depend on how much time and effort you invest. As with any project, you will get out of it what you put in.

Where do you start?

Have you tried it all before and none of it worked? Let me ask you, what if you did things differently? What if you made some changes just for a day and then found you could make them again the next day? Would that prove to you that if you can do it for a day, you can do it for a week? Soon, that week will turn into a month, and that month will turn into two months, and then a year. Then you have lasting and sustainable change. I am not asking you to do anything I have not done myself, and trust me when I tell you that if I can do it, then so can you.

My beliefs have changed over the years and now if I want something, I go for it. I don't waste time dabbling, I know that once I've made the decision to do something, I can do it – this can be true for you too. If you set your sights on making these changes happen and step across the line, you will discover that you have the ability to change in more ways than you ever thought possible. When you fix in your mind that you will make changes and that you will succeed, the process becomes a lot easier. Real health begins in the mind and making that mental decision is a must – there is no way around it. I want to encourage you to make the decision to improve your health and inspire you to take control.

Let's focus on helping you identify the steps that you need to concentrate on in order to create your own tailor-made prog-ramme. As you gradually adjust, you can decide when you're ready to move on to the next stage. This approach will make it so much easier to incorporate these steps into your life and help you sustain them over a longer period of time. Remember, this is not a quick fix. Changes that take place slowly and at a steady pace last a lot longer than those that occur overnight.

Most people find that the hardest part is making the decision to change in the first place, as most of us don't like change. We think we can't do it. Well, it's time to stop thinking about what you can't do and focus on what you can do. If you want to succeed, you need to identify what is standing in your way. For the vast majority of people, it is fear – fear of failing, which is possibly based on a past disappointment. But the fact is that we can learn valuable lessons from failure. So what if you fail? You can always try again. Remember we learn to walk by falling. Thomas Edison made many attempts at inventing the electric light bulb before he succeeded and with each attempt, he learned from his mistakes and turned his failures into success.

As most of us have no formal education in nutrition, it is so easy to ignore the impact that food has on our health. We have a fair idea about the principles of healthy eating but, somehow, we are often at a loss when we try to put this knowledge into practice. We are brainwashed by advertising that says we need dairy, meat and all manner of processed foods. Some doctors tell their patients that the foods they eat have nothing to do with the diseases they complain about, despite the scientific evidence to the contrary.

Do you believe that bad food can make you sick? If so, do you also believe that good, nutritious foods can nourish and heal your body? These questions are not just good discussion points, they are areas that need to be addressed if we are all to achieve good health. I hear people talking about how someone was 'very unlucky with their health' or how it was dreadful that somebody had a heart attack/stroke/cancer as 'they never drank or smoked'! But there is a much bigger picture to consider than just cigarettes and alcohol. Of course, they are not good for us, but we also need to be practical about the food we eat each and every day and the lifestyle choices we make.

There has never been a time when we have had so much inform-ation about health and yet my experience has shown me that the majority of people don't fully understand what makes their body tick. You would think that we would have a fair knowledge about what the correct foods to eat are, given the flood of information on the internet, TV programmes and, dare I say, the tons of books available on what a balanced diet should contain. Yet, many of us find it hard to face up to the reality that our physical wellbeing is largely dependent on the food we eat. It's easy to savour the nutritionally devoid food that has become the Western diet, but we are jeopardising our health when we eat foods that are not required by our bodies for normal healthy function. We can't afford to ignore this important fact if we are to create health for ourselves and our children.

Of course when illness strikes, it reminds us forcibly that we can no longer sidestep these issues. If you ever saw someone recovering from bypass surgery, I assure you that you would avoid unhealthy foods like the plague. Lifestyle, dietary and environmental factors need to be taken seriously.

With so many of our population falling prey to heart disease, diabetes and cancer, it is clear that something is drastically wrong with our eating patterns. More must be done to raise public awareness. Most people think that we need more drugs – or better drugs – to deal with these diseases, rather than addressing the causes of these illnesses.

I believe strongly that people are at a serious disadvantage when they don't understand what foods are needed to maintain their health. I always encourage my students to become informed, as this helps them when they are evaluating their options. Knowledge is power – but remember that knowledge is only effective when we put it into practice.

Clear information about food is so important, especially when you consider that every strand of DNA in us is made from nutrients and that every aspect of our body – literally and bio-logically – requires nutrition. I am convinced that if we focus on strengthening the body's immune system and ability to fight disease, we would all reduce our risks of being affected by cancer, heart disease and diabetes. Eating nutritious food is the most important health measure that any of us can take.

Most of the habits we develop around food are programmed into us from an early age. As a result, we often develop good or bad habits surrounding food without realising it. We grow up on the traditional Western diet of meat (including chicken), milk, fat, white bread and refined sugars. When I began to research the role foods play in influencing and inhibiting the promotion of disease, I came across a lot of research and case studies from doctors that showed the inextricable link between the food we eat and our overall health.

Doctors such as Dr Caldwell Esselstyn, a leading cardiologist, found that a plant-based diet not only prevents and stops the progression of heart disease, but can actually reverse its effects. In his book *Prevent and Reverse Heart Disease*, Esselstyn explains that eating meat and dairy injures the lining of our blood vessels, causing heart disease, heart attacks and strokes. He inspired the former American president Bill Clinton to move to a plant-based diet, which lead to Clinton's subsequently losing twenty-four pounds in weight. Many of Esselstyn's patients who had been given less than a year to live were symptom-free after only months on his diet.

Dr Colin T. Campbell, Professor Emeritus of Nutritional Bio-chemistry at Cornell University, explored the detrimental effects of eating animal foods. Contrary to many modern diets, Campbell uses scientific studies, mainly what became known as *The China Study*, to point out how nutrition influences our health and longevity. The scientific evidence he uncovered about the effects of diet on health had such a profound effect on him that he and his family changed to a 100 per cent plant-based diet. His message is clear – Western food causes Western diseases. He reports that most cancers are preventable and most heart-related conditions of arterial blockage and type 2 diabetes can be corrected by simply switching to a plant-based diet.

Another noteworthy figure is Dr Dean Ornish, the famous cardio-logist who pioneered the reversal of heart disease through diet, exercise and stress management. Ornish has had tremendous success in reversing arterial blockages of the heart without surgery or drugs. The people who participated in his lifestyle-intervention programme have had incredible results. He has the documented, clinical studies to back up his programme which has led to the reversal of coronary heart disease in his patients. Apart from practical steps and guidelines, Ornish also emphasises the value of love in health. In his book *Love and Survival*, he proposes that our very survival is also dependent on the healing power of love, intimacy and relationships.

Firmly rooted in science, the research from these eminent doctors has found that following a nutrient-dense, primarily plant-based diet can lower our risks of chronic diseases, such as heart disease, diabetes and cancer, and can help us to live longer, more vibrant and energetic lives.

Prevention is always better than a cure. It's cheaper, more effect-ive and, best of all, there is no risk involved. All research, even at the microbiological level, demonstrates the benefits of the prevention of disease – and prevention begins with you. If you emphasise preventative health care, you could substantially reduce your risk of contracting one of the many health problems that plague Western society. Certainly, we live longer today, but the truth is that the latter half of our lives is often stacked up with a host of health problems.

A question that is often posed is: 'Are we living longer or simply taking longer to die?'

I think most people would agree that living to a ripe old age is only something they would look forward to if they are active and independent to the end.

Becoming open to nutritional healing, opens up a world of alter-natives. Don't wait for a wake-up call before you employ some precautionary measures.

Another important element in making lifestyle changes is having a positive attitude, and there's a lot to be gained from realising this. Aligning your thoughts for change is an absolute necessity and is an important factor when it comes to food and lifestyle. Research by Dr Candace Pert, author of *Molecules of Emotion,* shows that positive, or negative, actions send messages to the body's immune system. She has published over 250 scientific articles, discussing how our brain, glands and immune system are in constant communication through emotions. Monocytes (key components of the immune system) have receptor sites for neuropeptides (information molecules), which link responses in the brain directly to the immune system. It seems our defence system is part of a complex network, linking our intellect, emotion and body, and not just an independent physical guard against disease. Remember that positive thinking is just as powerful as negative thinking. Your thinking plays a huge role in influencing you're eating patterns. This might seem like I am stating the obvious, but most people don't realise how important it is to be prepared for change and they jump in and expect the changes to work out. You are far more likely to succeed if you are positive, proactive and prepared. You need to have a plan before you start – this is an absolute must if you are to respond to change in a beneficial way. Your plan must be at the heart of every decision you make, and it will help enormously, especially during the first few weeks. Be clear about what you want to achieve. Do you want to lose weight? If so, how much? Do you want to clear up a health issue? If so, what steps are you prepared to take to sort out the problem? Do you want to teach your children healthy habits? If so, what do you want them to do differently? Are you going to get stuck in and sort it or are you going to dabble at sorting it out?

Your intention has to be clearly defined, otherwise you will be easily distracted. A plan will help you to manage the daily tasks and keep you focused on making a deliberate effort to take care of your health. Make a to-do list to help you get things done, if you have no experience of cooking or preparing foods, there are lots of simple recipes you can try (see Chapter 18 for some easy recipes to get you started). Start juicing, add nourishing foods to your daily regime and take some time out to go for a walk or do some exercise.

I am fortunate in that I get to see the progress that people make when they adopt a healthy lifestyle. Deirdre, a young woman who came to one of my three-day wellness programmes, had an experience I thought was worth sharing with you. The experience changed the framework of her life in ways she had not expected.

I am mailing to update you on how I've got on since the last programme in July. I had a fantastic time and learned so much over the weekend, a lot of which sits better with me than forcing myself to eat meat and eggs even though I don't like them. I loved the raw food that weekend and always cleared my plate and the juices were lovely, so I was off to a good start that I loved the fresh food.

Since then I have incorporated a few changes into my life for the better.

- I have given up dairy completely, which was easier than I thought.
- I have given up meat and eggs (anything with a mother or a face).
- I have been taking Udo's Oil which I love. My skin and hair are thanking me for it. It is great.
- I have my (non-dairy) smoothies every day.
- I'll never use a microwave again.
- My phone no longer stays in my bedroom and is switched off at 11 p.m.
- I am using natural soap and shampoos.
- I make the pumpkin spelt bread and everyone loves it now.

- I am trying to add a new thing every week.
- I cannot wait to get a juicer.

I feel I have more energy and concentration already, so I can't imagine how great it'll be to incorporate juicing to this.

My skin looks better and my face looks healthier, which is great.

My PMS symptoms have greatly improved too – an added bonus.

I am still in the dabbler stage, but am on the road to fully embracing the lifestyle change for sure. I was told by two dieticians and numerous doctors to eat sweets and frys and full-fat milk to help me bulk up, which would help my blood pressure stay up so I wouldn't feel faint but this just led to sugar highs and dips – you were right. Since I have stopped the sugar cycle, I am full without the sudden sugar dips and hunger. I didn't trust my body when I was getting vertigo and sugar dips but now I am feeling healthy in my body and feel I have nothing to worry about. Thanks a million for sharing your message. It's truly inspirational.

Far from dabbling at these changes, Deirdre made impressive progress in just one month. She came to my programme to make a few improvements to her eating habits and found that these lifestyle changes are not just about food but they are enriching, valuable and life-enhancing in more ways than one. These simple changes created a domino effect in her life. You, too, can make these simple changes – make them for a month and, as the benefits multiply, you won't go back.

Key points to remember

- Set yourself a target, it will help you to stay focused on your goal. Remember if you don't have a clear intention, you only have a dream.

- Lead from the front. Your example may influence others especially when they see the energy levels you are enjoying. If you pass on the practical changes you have learned, you might inspire others to improve their health.

- Don't let doubts block your progress. When you cast doubt on the steps you're trying to make, it dilutes your resolve. The more concentrated and focused you are, the fewer the doubts that will block your progress.

- Be consistent. Without consistency, you end up being side-tracked and drift away from your goal. If you are not consistent, it will be difficult to succeed in transforming unhealthy, addictive eating habits.

- Don't think too far ahead. Have a timescale for how long you will keep to your plan. Plan for a week and then turn a week into a month, and a month into a year.

- Educate yourself. There is a list of good reading resources by many eminent doctors at the end of this book.

- Go ahead and try it. You're worth it.

2

Getting your family on board

'The improvement of understanding is for two ends: firstly, our own increase of knowledge; secondly, to enable us to deliver that knowledge to others.'

JOHN LOCKE

Sometimes when I talk to people, I realise that we share the same problems and are faced with the same struggles. None of us is alone in trying to get our family members to improve their health. It is something that many of us struggle with – the fussy toddler, a grumpy teenager, even the husband or wife who is set in their ways.

At the risk of being ostracised by my family, I would like to share with you some of the successes and failures we have experienced since I started trying to change their eating habits.

When I was diagnosed with cancer for a second time, I wanted to improve not just my own health but also the health of my husband and children. At that stage, my daughter Julie was five years old and I had two teenagers – Sarah aged sixteen and Richard aged nineteen – and my husband Ger, who had no intention of changing his ways.

When you learn about the dangers that eating certain foods can bring, and how those foods can escalate health problems, you want to do what you can to avoid them. I must say it was not easy trying to get my family on board. In fact, I was surprised by how stuck in their ways they actually were. My efforts to improve their health caused a tremendous amount of conflict at meal times. Believe me, I learned many valuable lessons as I navigated my way through the conflict and friction.

My husband Ger is a firm believer in 'a little of what you fancy does you good', and many of us cling to this type of social conditioning. Ger tends to be a very task-focused, hands-on person who has a talent for getting things done. Yet, there was no way that he was prepared to expend time or energy needed to give up his favourite foods. This was despite the fact that he had developed arthritis and had high cholesterol, which his doctor had advised him to get under control or risk suffering a heart attack. The doctor had prescribed cholesterol-lowering drugs, anti-inflammatories and referred Ger to a specialist.

At that time, I was researching for one of my books and had just read a study in the *Archives of Internal Medicine* by Dr E. Cho of Harvard Medical School, which stated that taking non-steroidal, anti-inflammatory drugs increased the risk of kidney cancer by 50 per cent. Even more alarmingly, the study indicated that for the long-term users of these drugs (for ten years or more), the risk of developing kidney cancer tripled. Ger's specialist did explain to him that the anti-inflammatories she had prescribed may cause more serious side-effects and that he would be required to have his liver function checked every six weeks.

It seemed that he was in a no-win situation. Was he to take the drugs and risk further damaging his health? Or was he to continue suffering debilitating pain?

I did not want him to subject his body to either of these options.

You might think that this information would have inspired a turnaround from Ger, but he was not ready to throw off the habits of a lifetime even though, deep down, he knew he was short-changing his health. He knew that he needed some changes to his lifestyle because of his various health issues, but he was convinced that he only needed a few small adjustments – like taking some vitamin C pills and a few multivitamins to ensure that he covered any deficiencies in his diet. That was as far as he was prepared to go. If he could grab a few magic bullets and keep the old bad habits alongside, that would be the ideal quick fix.

He was not alone in his desire for a magic bullet, it is something that resonates with many of the people I help. People search for one therapy that will help them recover, whether it is the latest vitamin pill or a new scientifically proven drug. I have seen people take all manner of alternative treatments and concoctions in the hope that they will find the one treatment that will heal them *and* allow them to continue with their existing diet and lifestyle. Equally, I have first-hand experience of (as well as having witnessed many others suffer) the dramatic side-effects from medical treatments and pharmaceutical drugs. A complete recovery of physical and emotional health has to involve good food, an active lifestyle and a good mental outlook.

In light of his doctor's warnings, I felt the time had come for Ger to wake up and not continue down the road of self-sabotage. He could no longer take his health for granted. He needed to take charge of the situation and invest some effort into finding a way to improve his situation.

In a bid to get Ger to identify the habitual, negative choices he was making and start to eliminate them from his diet, I explained that he had to look at what he was eating. I did not want him to rely entirely on the medical establishment to deal with his health issues as they had offered him nothing but drugs, which I felt was merely putting a band-aid over the problem.

I tried hard to persuade him and hoped that he would come round to my way of thinking. As I saw it, he had a choice as relying on strong drugs with invasive side-effects was not the only option available to control his symptoms. Ger, on the other hand, was adamant that I should not fuss and dismissed my suggestions of a new dietary regime. He couldn't see the sense in it and, anyway, he was far too busy. You may want your loved ones to change to give them a better life, but if they are not open to it, your efforts will produce poor results. For some, the motivation factor has to be big in order to bring about lifestyle change.

I was unwavering in my resolve to help him avoid an inexorable slide into taking prescription drugs and was determined to do everything in my power to help him. As I believe strongly that food has healing benefits as well as nutritional ones, I made sure that he ate only organic food. I also began juicing for him regularly, I put him on a good supplementation regime and, above all, I did my best to appeal to his taste buds. After some time, he experienced a drop in his cholesterol-levels and his painful arthritis diminished. Who says you cannot teach an old dog new tricks!

The encouragement from this small victory was the incentive I needed to sort out the kids. One change can often pave the way for another and when you pile one success on top of another, you soon realise that change creates its own momentum. It is better to make one change than to do nothing at all.

Firstly, I cleared out the fridge and cupboards of all processed foods – believe me, they were not happy campers, but it meant that they were eating healthily by default as there were no treats or junk food in the house to munch on. I'll admit that there was a bit of friction initially as they did not want their comfort zone disrupted. It is fairly common to experience hostility in these situations. I am afraid that's human nature.

Every parent wants to provide the best for their children and conflict was the last thing I wanted during that transition period because I knew it would be counter-productive. In the face of this opposition, I learned to develop some sneaky tactics. I added essential fats in the form of oil to mashed potatoes, I put probiotic powder and raw vegetables into their smoothies and they never even noticed. I would love to report that these changes inspired them to change their eating habits but, to be honest, I had limited success with my teenagers. It's a difficult age.

My greatest triumph was with our five-year-old daughter Julie, who was still at an age where it was easy to influence her eating habits. Young children have not been brainwashed by advertising and have fewer preconceived notions about food. She was eager to learn and I encouraged her enthusiasm all the way. Julie became very clued in about eating healthy foods. As she embraced different elements of changing her eating habits, we focused on the foods she could eat (as opposed to what she couldn't). Every time she fancied a piece of chocolate or had cravings for sweets, I gave her healthy treats in exchange for the ones she normally liked. This simple tactic changed the way she ate.

Her enthusiasm was infectious. She was like a sponge for knowledge and I taught her which foods helped the different parts of her body. I tried to add a sense of adventure to her meals by introducing new foods. She enjoyed picking out interesting-looking fruit and vegetables while we were shopping and she found a few favourites to add to our healthy repertoire. All of these things gave her a healthy attitude towards food. At ten years of age, Julie decided to become a vegetarian and initially was concerned that her friends would tease her. The last thing she wanted was to stand out from the crowd. It turned out that her friends were very accepting of her preference to avoid meat and now they no longer comment on it. Julie has a few treats every now and then but I have to say she has exceeded my expectations for someone so young.

Encourage and educate – but don't nag

If you are trying to change the eating habits of your family, be prepared for disappointments and don't become disheartened.

You will almost certainly encounter some difficulties, so remember a few basic things. If your cupboards are full of junk food that they can snack on, then that is exactly what will happen. A fussy toddler sometimes needs to be hungry in order to eat proper meals. Instead of taking a firm stance and battling every day of the week with children, get them involved in some task when you are preparing a meal or snack, for example washing veggies, whisking a sauce or stirring a pot.

Children are far more likely to eat something that they have helped to make and it's a great time to fill them in on little bits of information about the foods they are eating. It's also good training, and children are much more adventurous with food when they prepare it themselves. When they learn about which foods nourish the body, they gain a better understanding of how to feed themselves. Building an understanding fosters awareness and responsibility. Your efforts *will* be rewarded.

Puberty is a natural process but if you have teenagers who are sometimes like bears ready to bite your head off, it might be worth looking at the foods they are eating. The underlying causes of these sudden shifts in hormonal balance are often based in physical changes.

When the sex hormones oestrogen, progesterone and testosterone are out of balance, it causes fatigue, irritability, fuzzy thinking, fluctuating emotions and PMS. These hormones are important neurotransmitters in the brain and deficiencies in nutrients can cause an imbalance in brain chemistry. The brain, like all other organs in the body, needs optimal nutrition.

Ups and downs are often triggered by too much sugar and a lack of essential fats such as flax, sunflower or sesame oils (see more on this on page 65). Often teenagers don't understand why they are irritable and snappy, and it is a relief to them and their parents to know that these symptoms can be alleviated if they eat different foods. Mood swings can be very difficult to deal with, however overreacting to outbursts can sometimes make things worse. Stay calm, reduce their sugar intake and add good fats to their diet in order to reduce angry or impatient flare-ups.

Even adults can suffer from mood swings. It's well known that sugar causes high and low blood-sugar levels. This constant roller-coaster means your unfortunate body is faced with the challenge of trying to restore a state of equilibrium. Essential fats elevate your mood and can lift depression. I have lots of readers who have been very successful at relieving severe mood swings by reducing their sugar intake and increasing the essential fats in their diets.

If you want to motivate teenagers, remember that they are very interested in how they look, so slip in bits of information about what foods help clear spots, keep them slim, eliminate period pains and give them energy. Believe me, it works wonders. If weight is their main focus, point out how many footballers, rugby players and athletes live on this food in order to perform to their best.

Encourage and welcome any interest your teenagers show, don't preach to them as they usually switch off if you start nagging about eating properly. It's admirable that you want to right the wrongs, but it could be to your detriment. I know it's not easy without their support, and it would be nice if you felt supported in your choice to get the family to eat more healthily, but you may have to rein in your urge because teamwork is not always the reality. I am all for getting children to think through and evaluate their decisions, but the fact remains that they may not always make the connection that the food that goes into their mouths has a direct bearing on their health.

If your children told you that they didn't want to brush their teeth any more, you wouldn't give them a choice. You would probably ignore their protests or explain why it's necessary. Meal times can become a battlefield that descends into pleading with them to eat their veggies or promising treats if they eat up. Kids don't have to love everything they eat. Sometimes they need to understand that it is good for them and that not eating it is not an option.

It's up to you as parents to set new standards if you don't like the way they are eating. Expect them to eat fruit and veg each day. Hand them pieces of veg while you are chopping or leave little tubs in front of them if they are playing or watching TV. Instead of treating food as a reward for good behaviour, change to offering them treats of going to the park, a trip to the zoo or have some friends over to play. The promise of a trip to the cinema or a day out shopping works well for teenagers.

Don't expect them to take it all on board immediately. They will come back to you for information when it becomes relevant to them.

However, if you are the one preparing food for the family, you need to take the initiative and take charge of the task. Always acknowledge results. It's the best way to get things done and bring your ideas to fruition.

Key points to remember

- Make a start – you have to make a deliberate effort to take care of your children's health (and that of other members of your family). Change is not going to happen out of the blue. Don't wait for the right time, the time is right now.

- Start slowly, introduce changes one meal at a time. If you push them too much initially, they are likely to rebel.

- Don't make any big announcements that the family has to change its ways, because that is likely to end in confrontation. A gentle, no-nonsense approach works better.

- If you end up with a revolution on your hands, have a contingency plan to get sneaky. It worked for me.

- Find healthy substitutes. There are lots of products that are good alternatives to your regular food choices. Cow's milk can be substituted with rice, oat or almond milk. Sugar can be substituted with stevia, and dairy butter with almond or hazelnut butter.

- Add good foods to your diet, because a nourished body tends to have fewer cravings.

- Be strong when they are weak. If they have a bad day and deviate from your plan get them back on track as soon as possible.

- Once you introduce a change, stick with it until it becomes ingrained into your daily routine.

- Remember it's not an all-or-nothing situation. It is better to make one change than do nothing at all.

3

Becoming a discerning shopper

'We cannot solve our problems with the same thinking we used when we created them.'

ALBERT EINSTEIN

It may sound like a chore to read the ingredients of the foods that you are putting into your shopping basket, but reading labels can help you make smart food choices. The foods we eat today are often far removed from their original natural state and can be highly processed and globally produced. The modernisation that occurred during the twentieth century brought about the widespread use of chemical fertilisers, pesticides, herbicides, additives, preservatives and other contaminants. Although these developments reduced food shortages, they have also had a negative effect on our health.

Most of us have tunnel vision when it comes to food, but let's not beat about the bush here – the fact is that many of the foods that are eaten today not only lack nourishment but also contain harmful ingredients. If we become complacent and cut corners with our health, how long will it take before our bodies decide it's payback time?

The problems associated with the mass production of food cannot be ignored. Food production today is based on economics not health. Our eating patterns may be strongly linked to habit and emotions, but they are also strongly linked to advertising. Mass marketing clearly uses psychology to promote and sell products. Some foods that are labelled 'healthy option', 'healthy choice', 'healthy alternative', etc. should possibly be labelled 'buyer beware'. Maybe it is time to open our eyes to what is really on offer. Despite the fact that you buy these products in good faith, you need to keep in mind that the desire for profit is the motivating force behind much of the food that is available for sale.

Although the advertisers' agenda is to make us buy their products, maybe not everything is their fault – maybe we have got it wrong. Perhaps we don't want to take on board the health issues these foods can bring because we can't bear the thought of going without familiar foods like sugar, dairy products and fatty foods, even though we know our health pays a high price when we eat them.

Every time we buy food, we make a choice. Consumers wield economic power and an educated and aware population should encourage the production of foodstuffs that will protect health, not endanger it. There is real potential for consumers to create healthy change to advance a healthy society. As demand increases for foods that are not irradiated, or laden with pesticides, herbicides, food colourings, artificial sweeteners, sugar, salt, synthetic hormones, and growth and appetite stimulants, food producers may have to readjust their profit margins.

When you begin to read labels, you discover some unsavoury truths about the common foodstuffs we have been weaned on. Even a diligent consumer who continually checks labels would need a chemistry degree to decipher the list of ingredients in some products. Don't assume that the products that line the shelves in shops are automatically good for you, it is up to you to check the list of ingredients. I recently checked out what I thought were healthy savoury crackers in my health store only to find they were laden with sugar.

When taking a closer look at the ingredients here are some things to watch out for:

- *'Fortified', 'enriched', 'added' and 'extra'*: These are all terms used by manufactures to encourage you to buy their products. What they often mean is that vitamins, minerals and fibre have been removed during processing – food producers must add artificial supplements to replace the natural ones they have removed. It is nearly impossible to find any fortified food product that does not contain some form of synthetic vitamins, and synthetic vitamins are just more chemicals.

- *'Sugar-free' and 'fat-free'*: This can mean that the manufacturer has had to compensate with other ingredients to ensure consistency and taste, but those ingredients may have the same number of calories as the sugar and fat that have been left out. This has led to people not only avoiding sugar but replacing it with heavily processed alternatives that really are no healthier.

- *'Natural'*: Some food products are marketed to 'prevent' health conditions. Thousands of processed food products are promoted in this way. Processed foods cannot replace the vast range of nutrients and phytochemicals that are present in foods in their original natural state.

- *'Wholegrain' and 'wholewheat'*: Using the word 'whole' has led to an incorrect assumption that these products are effective in promoting health. These products are produced on a massive commercial scale and may have very little wholegrain left in them after processing. In the USA, state governments have made it mandatory that white flour is artificially enriched with crystalline B vitamins, niacin and iron, and synthetic vitamins are added into many of our breads, cereals and other grain products.

- *'Organically grown', 'pesticide-free' and 'no artificial ingredients'*: Have you ever wondered if you can trust organically grown foods? Trustworthy growers work hard to attain their certification and their fruits and vegetables are consistently tested for pesticide residue. Only buy foods that are certified organically grown and have a certification number to prove it on the label.

Think about it, what makes more sense – pesticides, herbicides, fungicides, chemical fertilisers, artificial additives and high-fructose corn syrup or organic, natural food from Mother Nature? It does not take a scientist to work out which is better for your health.

Key points to remember

- Make a shopping list. Planning is essential, otherwise you could be tempted by special offers and influenced by product placement rather than what you need to buy. The grocery store can be a place of constant temptation. Stick to your list and you will be more likely to make healthy choices.

- Avoid shopping when you are hungry. Hunger-fuelled shopping is disastrous as you will often be guided by your hunger pangs not your health.

- Do yourself a favour as you make your way through the supermarket, dodge the aisles with chocolate, biscuits, crisps and soft drinks. It is likely to lead to impulse buying.

- When looking at labels, check for added sugars such as corn syrup, cane juice, dextrose, lactose, glucose, maltose, fructose and malt syrup. Nearly a quarter of additional calories come from added sugars.

- Remember that products with long lists of ingredients are usually full of preservatives. These foods have the potential to put your health at risk.

- Steer away from foods with hydrogenated fats. If you see 'trans-fats' on the list of ingredients, don't buy the product.

- Move to more whole foods and buy foodstuffs that don't use ingredients you are not familiar with.

- Most meal plans become monotonous after a while – try and mix things around every few weeks.

- As a rule of thumb, trust your gut instincts and make smart choices.

4

Eating organic food on a budget

'Good food is wise medicine.'

ALISON LEVITT MD

Most people assume that they will pay hugely inflated prices for organic foods, however, even if you are on a tight budget, you can eat organically. Your meals can be almost 100 per cent organic if you organise yourself with a carefully thought-out shopping list. Planning meals may seem tedious, especially when so many processed foods are readily available, but having a plan will keep you in control of your budget as well as ensuring your health.

People often ask me if it is worth spending extra money on organic produce, and my answer is always YES. Especially when you consider the long-term dangers of pesticides are neurological symptoms, immune systems disorders, liver disease and asthma attacks. Can we honestly believe that there is no threat to our health if our bodies' resources are spent trying to rid us of chemicals from food?

Recently one of my friends, who is quite interested in health and who has made great progress in changing her eating habits, questioned me about buying or not buying organic foods. I explained that in the past 50 years alone, 3,500 more individual chemicals have been added to the foods we eat. She had assumed that our foods were not harmful and that the government wouldn't allow foods that could harm us to be sold here. We discussed the dangers associated with eating chemically sprayed foods and how it was not good economic sense to eat foods that could promote the development and progression of disease.

I asked her why she would not take the next step and move to organic foods, given that she was so close to getting her eating habits right. She said that while she understood the concept and reasoning behind what I was saying, she could simply not justify the extra cost and was not prepared to scrutinise every purchase she made. One point worth noting is that if the emphasis in the market place was on safe, nutritious food, our buying decisions would be based on health and not on saving money. As we discussed the economics of the weekly shopping bill versus the cost to the health of the family and soaring health costs, I realised that, for my friend, it was more about the effort it would take to check what she was eating rather than the cost of organic foods. I understand it can be overwhelming initially to read labels but remember your health is at stake.

After some gentle prodding from yours truly, she began to take the time to check the labels of the foods she was eating. Together we devised a list of a few things she could monitor in her shopping. She made quite a few adjustments to her weekly shopping list when she became aware of the ingredients in the foods she had been eating. Label reading does not have to take a long time and you will quickly become familiar with the healthier brands and where to source them.

All the pesticides and chemicals that are being sprayed onto our foods end up on our plates. I always recommend that people who are curious about eating organic foods should answer a question: if they picked an apple from a tree in their garden, would they spray it with a chemical before they ate it? This usually ends the debate for those who still think there is a debate. If you want to take care of your health, why not choose the healthiest, safest food available?

I no longer approach chemically sprayed food products from the price tag they carry but instead from the knock-on effect they have on my health. I am not prepared to trade-off my health to save money as I believe it is a false economy, particularly if you end up paying out exorbitant fees on medical care and treatments. You need to be conscious about what is going into your mouth if you want to maintain a healthy body. Be observant and be wary of chemically sprayed foods.

The good news is that you get to choose. Adopting a healthy diet can save money at the same time as boosting your health. Visit your local farmers' market – I find they are sometimes susceptible to a bit of persuasion and give better deals on organic produce. Also when crops are plentiful, they are likely to cost less, so buy in season if you're trying to reduce your weekly budget. We are all influenced by a bargain, but cheap foods that contain harmful substances are not the answer.

Grow your own

If you still think that organic vegetables are too expensive to buy, why not grow your own? A lot of vegetables can be grown in pots or small beds in your garden and seeds are very cheap. If you have a few feet of space to grow things why not try it? Trust me when I tell you I am no gardener but I have made significant savings on my groceries each week since I started growing vegetables and salad leaves in my back garden. I have grown lettuces and tomatoes for years and recently bought a small raised bed. I take all my kitchen vegetable waste and put it into a large size compost bin full of earthworms so I have my own compost which helps me grow kale, lettuces, spring onions, chives and Swiss chard. I chose these because they only take a few weeks to grow from seed. It's lovely picking the veg and juicing it straight away, much more nourishing than the week old, wrinkled specimens in the bottom of the fridge, and so much better for you as you don't lose the nutrients.

Don't assume growing vegetables is complicated. You will be surprised how quickly your garden will supply you with many wonderful things to eat. A garden is not just for pleasure and you can turn even the smallest space into a useful place to grow a few vegetables and herbs. Growing your own food is very rewarding, as well as being healthy, and the vegetables taste much better because they have not spent days on the shelf in a supermarket deteriorating. The longer you food is on the shelf, the more nutrients it loses.

With the downturn in the economy, there has been a big resurgence in the number of people 'growing their own'. It's become the 'in thing'. A farmer close to me has rented his field as allotments, and gives all the money he receives to charity. It's really heart-warming to see so many people of all ages reconnecting with nature and gaining such a positive outcome. There are community gardens if you don't have space for a garden – check out www.giyireland.com.

If you are looking for an instant vegetable garden, there are companies that supply kits which include a compost mix and a tray of baby vegetable plants that are ready to just pop into the soil. Some companies deliver straight to your door (see the Resources section). They have free video tutorials on their websites and lots of other helpful information to make sure people who want to get into growing have a successful experience. Your garden will be an instant success.

If getting out in the air to grow your own food is food just not your style, why not try growing some sprouted beans and seeds indoors? It's a good way to save money and there are amazing benefits to be gained from growing your own sprouts. Sprouts are the baby plants in their prime, such as cress, alfalfa, fenugreek, broccoli and sunflowers. I do not mean Brussels sprouts. One lady juiced Brussels sprouts for months before she realised her mistake. I can't imagine how her juice must have tasted. Yuck!

According to experts, the sprouting stage in the development of plants is the time when they have the largest concentration of proteins, vitamins, minerals, enzymes and bioflavonoids. Not only are they a fantastic source of food and nutrients, they are also economical. Sprouts are living foods. These wholesome, nutritious foods are constantly growing right up until the time of consumption. The Hippocrates Health Institute in Florida uses sprouts as part of its therapeutic programme for treating all kinds of diseases, such as cancer, heart disease and arthritis. This is because of the amazing healing powers and anti-cancer properties these baby plants have. Sprouts contain the most concentrated natural source of enzymes, vitamins and minerals and amino acids which are vital for a healthy body.

You do not need any soil or much space to grow these powerful healing foods because they can be grown indoors in jars. These little seedlings have stored within them the nourishment to support a fully grown plant. If you have ever grown sunflowers you will know how one small seed can turn into a six-foot plant.

Seeds and grains do not grow without moisture but, once you add water, you activate their dormant enzymes – a massive enzyme release occurs as the seed springs to life. As they begin to grow, they release vitamin C and a flood of vitamins (including vitamins A, B-complex, C, D and E). Sprouts are packed full of proteins, iron, enzymes calcium, potassium, magnesium, amino acids and essential fatty acids. They are so simple to grow and a small handful of seeds will yield a good crop of sprouts in about two to four days, so they are ready to eat in a short timeframe.

They are great value for money when you consider their many benefits. They can be added to salads, soups, sandwiches and juices. Sprouts boost the immune system and protect us against disease. Small children grow watercress sprouts in school in egg cups, so if little kids can do it – so can you. It only takes about five minutes a day to grow these nutritious foods. Give it a go as there is nothing more rewarding than growing your own food.

Learning how to produce a regular supply of organic sprouts can be a wonderful boost to your budget and health, especially when you consider the dangers of the toxic chemicals in many of today's foods. If you really don't want to grow them, they can also be bought in many stores, supermarkets, health food stores and online.

Rest assured, you really can eat organic foods on a budget.

Key points to remember

- Visit your local farmers' market and buy foods that are in season.

- Try growing your own. You will be saving money and you will literally be growing your own organic vegetables! You don't need green fingers, it's really quite simple when you water a seed it grows, and Mother Nature does the rest. Also grow your own sprouted beans and seeds, indoors in jars.

- Organic foods are no longer difficult to find. Today, there are more and more organic products in the grocery store. Even the large chain stores are selling organic produce. But remember to check their certification number.

- If you spend money on organic foods, don't destroy their nutritional benefits by putting them into a microwave.

5

Convenience versus nourishment

'Insanity is doing the same thing over and over again and expecting different results.'

ALBERT EINSTEIN

D o you believe that 'you are what you eat' or, more importantly, 'what you absorb'? Yes, it's true, what you put into your body has a direct bearing on your health and your weight. As our health is based on the amount of absorbable nutrition we provide to our bodies, it would seem that it is necessary to get back to some grass-root solutions if we are to solve the problems that result from nutritionally poor diets.

I grew up in the era where my mother picked vegetables from the garden, baked her own bread and prepared everything that fed our family. Today, all that has changed. People appreciate convenience foods, but it is so difficult to garner similar support for freshly prepared foods. Some people only really eat convenience foods, and buy a lot of pre-packaged, ready-to-cook, ready-to-heat and ready-to-eat foods to save preparation time.

It is extremely challenging to try and eat healthily if you are struggling to keep up with everyday life. It can be difficult to make time for all that chopping, peeling or steaming and many people find it is much easier to reach for the unhealthy option. Okay, these foods are quick and easy to dish up and certainly more convenient than meals made from scratch with fresh ingredients, but they are not going to give you and your family the nourishment you need to look and feel great.

I have voiced my apprehension time and time again about convenience foods because eating these foods can be a hazard to your health. As we become more educated about what exactly is in the convenience foods we are eating and become more health conscious, we are waking up to the fact that food manufacturers are now selling ready-meals in the guise of health foods.

Take, for example, white bread. Most people know that brown bread is more nutritious than white bread. This is because to produce white flour the bran and the germ are removed from the whole-wheat grain during the refining and bleaching process. Fibre, vitamins, minerals and trace elements are lost, and the bread must then be fortified with synthetic nutrients to replace the natural nutrients that have been removed. It sounds crazy to take away naturally occurring nutrients and then put back 'artificial nutrients', but such is the madness of convenience foods.

Shelf life should also be taken into consideration if you want to avoid foods that are laden with additives and preservatives. Always read the ingredients list and stay away from foods that contain ingredients you don't recognise.

A few years ago, I asked a group of students (who ranged from 25 to 58) if they ate a well-known make of white bread rolls. Every person in the group had eaten these rolls, for most they were a basic staple of their weekly diet. So I decided to conduct a few experiments on bread rolls, muffins and croissants to see how long they would last before decay or moulds developed on them. I bought them in my local store and I was astonished to find out how long they lasted.

I now have various rolls dating back to 2010 and muffins dating back to 2006, none of which show any sign of deterioration, apart from going hard. Imagine what preservatives were used to protect these foods from decay if they can last for seven years. I show these rolls and muffins at my seminars so people can see exactly how they have maintained their fresh look. We are often fooled by the freshly baked smell of these common staple foods and don't think that they contain preservatives and synthetic nutrients. Modern-day processed foods and labelling can be very deceiving.

There has been a gradual increase in the amount of organic produce available from farmers, but retailers will only get serious about organic food when consumers demand it. As long as there is a demand for processed convenience foods, that's what retailers will provide.

If you were to check your kitchen cupboards or freezer, how much of that food have you bought because of convenience and how much has been bought to nourish your body? You could pay a price for using foods that are stripped of nutrients and these short-sighted decisions can leave you susceptible to disease.

But don't panic. It is easy to stock your kitchen with healthy, convenient foods. If you realise that there are meals that can be prepared in a flash, you are more likely to succeed, and less likely to stick something in the microwave or send out for pizza.

You will have no problem incorporating 'healthy' food into your meals as soon as you begin to taste how delicious this food actually is. Once you get a feel for it, you will eat food of a far superior quality while also saving yourself some money.

In order to help eliminate poor food choices, I have always found it better to find alternatives and add them to the diet before eliminating those foods you are used to.

Adopting a healthy, plant-based diet

If you really want to play it safe, why not join the growing number of people moving to a plant-based diet? This may sound radical to those who have been raised on meat and fish – but just because we have eaten something for most of our lives, doesn't mean we have to carry on that way. It may seem difficult to get past the rigid thinking that we cannot survive without meat, but we can. I have not eaten any type of meat (and that includes chicken) or fish for over twelve years and my health has improved dramatically in that time. I promise you won't be living on a leaf of lettuce and a stick of carrot for dinner.

You may think a plant-based diet is just for health nuts, but think again. Many intellectual, athletic and successful people have adopted plant-based diets – Carl Lewis (Olympic champion), Albert Schweitzer (Nobel laureate), Biz Stone (co-founder of

Twitter) and Bill Clinton (former US president) to name just a few.

In 2004, Bill Clinton had quadruple bypass surgery and, some years later, had two stents put into his heart because his veins had clogged up once again. When he researched how to reverse his heart disease, he found that 82 per cent of the people who moved to a plant-based diet had cleared up their arterial blockages and reversed their heart disease. In the process of changing his diet, he also lost 24 pounds. He was happy to lose the weight but that was not his main objective. A previous lover of steaks and hamburgers, he no longer eats dairy products (including eggs), chicken, fish or other meat. Can you envisage what professional advice the ex-president of the USA must have had access to? Switching to a plant-based diet turned out to be a life-saver for Bill Clinton.

Adopting a healthy, plant-based diet can help you lose weight at the same time as boosting your health. Losing weight and staying slim are the obvious external payoffs for moving to a plant-based diet. After years of struggling to keep my weight in check, I discovered this myself when I switched after my second cancer diagnosis. While it was a welcome change, I was not excited for reasons of vanity. I knew from my research that the body doesn't heal selectively, and if my body was renewing and improving outwardly, then the same changes were taking place inside.

Albert Einstein once wrote:

> Nothing will benefit human health and increase chances for survival of life on Earth as much as the evolution to a vegetarian diet.

You might consider these words the next time you buy a steak. One of the problems with meat protein is that it is difficult to digest. Protein has to be broken down into amino acids to be beneficial, and high-protein foods require a massive amount of energy to break them down. To overcome the problem, your body must work overtime, struggling to digest proteins and this, in turn, puts added pressure on the immune system. In addition, undigested meat can remain in your intestines and become putrefied, and this leads to a toxic build up and often chronic ailments of the joints and heart set in.

While chicken is not as dense as beef or pork, it has its own problems. A lot of people eat lighter meats like chicken because they believe they are a healthier option. What they don't realised is that chicken can also raise LDL levels of 'bad' cholesterol.

We need to eat protein in a digestible form of amino acids. A plant-based diet is a much healthier option than one based around meat and fish. If you are not inclined to give up your daily portion of flesh, then try to add one vegetarian meal per week. Stick with this for a few weeks until it becomes the norm and then introduce a second vegetarian meal. Gradually adding a new dish on one or two days a week will enable your taste buds to adjust. My husband is a meat-eating man who is not prepared to give it up. I found a small bit of restructuring worked well and gave him a few nights each week without meat, which gave his body gets a rest from digesting all that protein. There are lots of wonderfully tasty recipes to tempt you in the recipe section on page 172.

Where will I get my proteins if I don't eat meat?

This is probably the question I am asked most, and it makes me realise how little education most people have about the foods we eat. We know a little, but we don't know enough.

There are a lot of misconceptions and myths about proteins, so let's look at the facts. Most people believe that they will wither away if they don't get enough protein, when in fact too much protein is associated with a number of diseases – it can raise blood cholesterol levels, can cause a decline in kidney function and can increase the risk of calcium loss, which can lead to osteoporosis.

The facts are that protein deficiency is impossible if we meet our daily calorie needs. Our protein needs are stupendously easy to meet as the body only requires a very small amount. The World Health Organization (WHO) recommends that men and women obtain 5–11 per cent of their calories as protein. WHO also makes clear that around 97 per cent of people need less than this.

Babies need twice as much protein as adults, breast milk contains 3–5 per cent protein. So at a time when their developmental needs are at their highest, the perfect food for babies contains only small amounts. There is no other time in a person's life that they will double in size. The simple fact is when you eat fresh food, you get more than enough protein.

Dr Marion Nestle of the Department of Nutrition Food Studies and Public Health at New York University states:

> We never talk about protein anymore, because it's absolutely
> not an issue, even among children. If anything, we talk about
> the dangers of high-protein diets. Getting enough is simply a
> matter of getting enough calories.

Let me ask you if you know anyone with a protein deficiency. I strongly doubt it. Protein deficiency diseases, such as kwashiorkor or marasmus, are very rare except in countries where people are starving. The Centre for Disease Control in America states that protein deficiency is most common amongst people in impoverished communities of developing countries and in the elderly who do not meet their daily calorie needs. Consider also the millions of Asian people who live long and healthy lives on rice and vegetable diets. Think of gorillas, a close genetic relative to humans, who survive mostly on a raw, plant-based diet. With their large muscular structure, gorillas are most certainly not deficient in protein.

Humans cannot store protein in their bodies. If you ingest a surplus amount of proteins, your body works hard to break it down. Extra pressure is then placed on your digestive system to break down the accumulation of protein by-products. Focusing on one nutrient source does not supply the body with the full range of nutrients that a varied diet provides and which your body needs.

Very often when people first switch to a vegetarian diet, they load up on cheese and carbohydrates, but this isn't a balanced approach either. Processed dairy foods, in the form of cheese and yogurts, are also indigestible, and processed carbohydrates will be stored by the body as fat. If you focus on having a balanced approach and gaining nutrients from a broad variety of vegetables, you are *guaranteed* to look and feel great.

Good sources of absorbable protein are sprouted seeds, beans, grains and leafy green vegetables. Vegetables are 22 per cent protein, nuts and seeds are about 11 per cent, whole grains 13 per cent, and beans 28 per cent. Now that you know the facts, you will think about your protein needs in an entirely new way. Don't believe those who have not bothered to check the scientific evidence. The next time someone asks you where you get your proteins, you will know the exactly what to say.

Eat more living food

If you want to recharge your batteries, eat more raw, living food. Heating your food is not good for your health because cooked food causes an inflammatory response called leukocytosis (elevated number of white cells in the blood). When food is heated above 40 degrees, its molecular structure changes – oils turn carcinogenic and proteins, vitamins and live enzymes are destroyed in the cooking process. The Max Planck Institute in Leipzig has found that cooking denatures proteins, which means that our bodies have to work harder to assimilate these dead foods. Because any beneficial enzymes have been destroyed by cooking, the food is difficult to digest and provides very little nourishment.

Foods that are stripped of nutrients will not fuel your body. Rather, they will leave you with an exhausted immune system. The human body is a machine that needs the correct fuel, much like your car needs fuel, oil and water. Humans have a physiological need for vitamins, minerals and other organic nutrients and these nutrients need to be supplied regularly and in high enough quantities in order to maintain a healthy body. If you abandon the formula, you increase your chances of lowering your immune system, your main ally against disease.

When foods are not cooked, their nutrients remain intact and, more significantly, live enzymes – the most important part of our foods – are not destroyed. All cellular activity of life depends on enzymes and, without them, there would be no life. Enzymes stimulate the body's killer T-cells to destroy cancer cells. Cooking destroys enzymes and forces the body to produce more of its own enzymes, which are secreted by our pancreas, and this leaves little left over for disease-fighting activity.

Enzymes enhance longevity significantly, as they slow down free-radical damage. This is another great reason to eat more raw living foods. It is definitely worth making the effort to enjoy these delicious natural tastes that will provide your body with much more nutrition. As the saying goes, it's not the food in your life, but the life in your food that nourishes your body.

Keep healthy snacks at hand

Keep nuts and seeds at hand for healthy snacks, as they work well at keeping hunger at bay. Fruit is also perfect when you need a sugar hit, and you could have some vegetables and hummus for a savoury fix. There are various crackers available in health-food shops, such as spelt crackers and rice cakes (although these still need to be taken in moderation), which can replace biscuits.

If the thought of an uncooked meal does not appeal to you, why not invest in a dehydrator? This is a small machine that warms food slightly without destroying the nutrients and gives the finished dish the appearance of being cooked. They are inexpensive (see the Resources section on page 244) and you can make crisps, snacks, biscuits, crackers and main meals that have not been cooked or heated in oils. They will produce satisfying, tasty and enzyme-rich foods for yourself and your family.

Dehydrators are great if you have left over fruit, such as apples, pineapples or mango. Just slice the fruits, dip them in lemon juice to stop discoloration and pop them in the dehydrator. Try the kale crisps recipe on page 225, they are so easy to make, are not fried or heated in oils, and taste delicious. My daughter Julie often pitches in with a helping hand when I make crisps – kids always feel so proud of what they have made themselves. These are super healthy snacks if you get the munchies, watching television, sitting at your desk and are great for kid's lunchboxes. You can buy these crisps in some speciality stores but it is much more economical to make you own. I get great pleasure from watching my students enjoy these yummy treats and it is nice to see how it opens them up to many new tastes and ideas.

I have suggested delicious recipes in Chapter 18 for you to try – there is a whole section devoted to crisps and crackers, but you will need a dehydrator to make them. The recipes will provide meals for you and your family that are not depleted of the vital nutrients that are essential for a strong, healthy body. Don't be put off by the length of time it takes to dry food. The time is not spent preparing the food, it's just the length of time it takes to dry them. It's not like an oven that you have to watch and there is no risk of burning food in a dehydrator.

Key points to remember

- If you're stuck for time, have a freshly prepared juice or smoothie from your nearest juice bar. You will be spoiled for choice.

- If you fancy a quick lunch, fresh salads from the deli counter are an ideal healthy alternative to sandwiches and take-outs.

- Avoid microwave meals, they might be convenient but microwaves denature food. You may be getting the calories but the vitamins, minerals and proteins will have been destroyed.

- Ready-prepared meals are high in salts. Eating excess sodium can be harmful to people with hypertension or high blood pressure and causes fluid retention.

- Eat less bread, potatoes and pasta and add more veggies to your meals. This can help you drop a size in no time. Your plate is always healthier if it is filled with bright foods with texture. Switch to my no-calorie spaghetti (see page 219), it is filling and tastes delicious served with my no-cheese basil pesto (see page 233).

- Reduce the number of carbohydrates on your plate with my low-carb rice (see page 218), which can be served with my hot and spicy curry (see page 207).

- Dish up a side of spinach. It will fill you up so it's a great way to add volume to your meals without the calories. Spinach provides 40 per cent of your daily need for magnesium, which is crucial for calcium absorption.

- Cut out empty calories from soft drinks. Think of all the artificial sweeteners they contain. Chemical sweeteners in diet soft drinks acidify the body and cause you to retain fluids, giving a bloated appearance.

- Instead of using just lettuce, add spinach in your salads. Varying the textures can take the boredom out of salads.

- Increase your fibre intake by replacing all white-flour products with whole grains. Switch to breads baked with sprouted spelt, buckwheat, millet, amaranth or quinoa. These grains have little or no gluten (the protein which can cause digestive problems) and are highly nutritious.

- Keep some basic items on hand, such as fresh onions, garlic, salad greens, lemons, olive oil, canned chick peas, sweetcorn, coconut milk and beans. You can easily throw together a tasty meal that is chock full of nutrients.

- Soups are great to have on hand if you get the munchies. Add parsley, spinach and garlic at the end of cooking, so you won't destroy their nutrients and beneficial oils.

- Throw in some sprouted quinoa to soups just before you serve. It's rich in protein and once sprouted the protein is more easily digested.

- Stews and veggie bakes are heart-warming especially in cold weather. They are ideal for those wanting to incorporate vegetarian dishes into the family menu.

- Stay away from high-protein diets, too much protein is associated with a number of diseases.

- Above all make wise choices about the food you eat. What you do now will dictate your future.

6

Juicing is easy

'An ounce of conscious choice is worth a pound of good
fortune.'

JONATHAN LOCKWOOD HUIE

I've spent many years studying what works and what doesn't in
the field of health and weight loss and, of all the steps I teach
to improve health and help people lose weight, juicing is the one
that is the most effective. If you are looking for a quick pick-me-
up to overcome fatigue and a lack of energy, juicing will give you
that new lease of life you are looking for. Juicers are easy to shop
for and easy to use.

Before you buy a juicer, which I highly recommend, a very simple
way to start is to add some lemon juice to water and begin your
day with two glasses of this refreshing liquid. It's a great way to
start the cleansing and detoxing process. If you find it difficult
to drink this quantity of water, heat the water slightly and that
should do the trick.

Lemon juice not only adds flavour but it has many medicinal properties. Lemons are rich in vitamin C and also contain small amounts of niacin and thiamine. The vitamin C content of lemons not only helps to stave off colds, it is also very effective at dislodging phlegm from the lungs. In the digestive tract, lemon juice destroys worms, relieves constipation and prevents vomiting. Vitamin C is also very effective in calcium metabolism.

Use the skin of lemons as well as it is loaded with phytonutrients, but make sure the lemons are organic to avoid exposure to pesticides. Always remove the peel from other citrus fruits, such as oranges, grapefruits and nectarines, before juicing, as they have a bitter taste and their oils are difficult to digest. Jethro Kloss wrote in his book *Back to Eden*:

> The medicinal value of the lemon is as follows: It is an antiseptic or is an agent that prevents sepsis [the presence of pathogenic bacteria] or putrefaction [the decomposition of tissue]. It is also anti-scorbutic, a term meaning a remedy which will prevent disease and assist in cleansing the system of impurities.

Bet you didn't know a humble lemon could be so useful! Remember real health is not rocket science, it's sometimes very simple.

A new lease of life

Without doubt, juicing is a wonderful way to improve your health and it is exactly why so many natural healing centres around the world have used juicing as part of their regimes for many decades. Fresh fruits and vegetables play a huge role in improving our health and wellbeing, and have outstanding nutritional qualities.

The benefits of juicing are many. Depending on the fruits and vegetables you use, juices can have antioxidant and anti-inflammatory components, essential enzymes, and vitamins and minerals, which keep all kinds of ailments and diseases at bay and are very effective in enhancing the growth of healthy cells. The World Cancer Research Fund in London estimates that high fruit and vegetable intake may reduce cancer incidence by 64 per cent.

The main reason that this type of liquid nutrition is used to heal the body is because the fruits or vegetables have not been cooked. When fruit and vegetables are consumed in their natural state, their nutrients remain intact. On the other hand, if you boil, steam or zap the life out of what you eat in a microwave, you are consuming dead food with little or no nourishment. Foods that are stripped of their nutrients are not going to nourish your body.

A daily routine of juicing is easy to put into practice, as you don't need fancy instructions or ingredients. All you need is just some fresh fruit and vegetables, a good juicer and the commitment of time to making two juices each day. Take it from me, it is well worth the effort. If you are a beginner, you can start with mixed fruit and vegetable juices and, as you progress, you can gradually phase out the fruits in favour of the veggies. Vegetable juices are less taxing on blood-sugar levels – even natural fruits can spike blood sugars. You can change the recipes so you don't get bored, and use you own favourite flavours to mix things up a bit.

I am not at all keen on celery which is a good source of potassium but juicing it is a great way to sneak it into my diet. Juicing works wonders for fussy teenagers or toddlers by enabling you to give them vegetables and leafy greens that they would normally refuse to eat. With the addition of an apple, lemon juice and a little coaxing, you will be amazed how many vegetables you can get into them in two juices a day. If you still think they won't go for it, add a little stevia to sweeten the juice, you will be pleasantly surprised with its taste. Juicing will help you raise healthy children and keep infections, colds and flu at bay, which means fewer trips to the doctor and fewer days off school.

These days, I am literally putting half my garden into my juicer and, topped with a spritz of lemon and a bit of ice, the juice tastes fantastic. For two half-litre glasses of juice per day, you will need six to eight portions of fruits and vegetables. See my new mouth-watering recipes on page 172, they should inspire you to get juicing.

When you start juicing, you will wonder why you have waited so long to make your *own* fresh juices. You will feel the benefits almost immediately of this simple step.

Increased energy

Juices are great at boosting energy. They improve stamina and will give you the increased 'oomph' you need to live life to the fullest. If you are struggling to stay awake in the afternoon or are always feeling tired, then juicing is the answer to your problems. To help the body perform at its best, add two glasses of freshly made juice to your daily routine. I guarantee you will have sustained energy throughout the day with this delicious addition to your diet. Many people refrain from eating before a workout, but the body needs fuel to give it energy and staying power when we exercise. Juicing provides that much-needed boost of nutrients for increased stamina plus it hydrates the body. There is no better way to help you get up and go!

Weight loss

Juicing is a great low-calorie way to fill you up and help you stay slim. Juices that contain no fruits work best if you want to lose weight and you can add lemon or ginger to suit your taste buds. Certain juices help speed up your metabolism and detoxify your body, which makes losing weight quicker and easier than would otherwise be the case. You can also add some healthy fats which will ensure you burn fat. This will help turn your fat cells around, so that instead of taking fat into the cells, they release fat to be used for energy. Remember if you want to lose fat, you have to eat fat. Don't believe those 'fat phobic' people who think that fats add nothing but calories to your food. It is imperative to recognise the difference between good fats and bad fats (see more on good fats on page 65). Fresh juices will flush out your system of stored waste particularly when taken first thing in the morning. Most people have impaired digestion, so if you suffer with constipation, green juices will alleviate even the worst congested intestines. Try it you will love it!

Improved health

Let's not forget that another major advantage of juicing is improved health. Juices have high concentration of highly absorbable nutrition. In just two juices a day, you can easily consume large quantities of fruits and vegetables, and your five-(to-ten)-a-day can be reached easily. The National Cancer Institute in America claims that we need nine to ten portions of fruit and vegetables each day, rather than the more usual five-a-day guideline (see www.cancer.gov). Consuming fruits and vegetables can reduce the occurrence of breast cancer by 31 per cent. When you get to see and feel the difference of this simple step to better health, you will realise how it revolutionises your body's ability to heal itself and boost your natural defences. Because of their therapeutic properties and amazing healing powers, juices are especially useful for people who are facing a health challenge. This highly concentrated form of liquid nutrition will give you the vitamins, minerals, enzymes and trace elements to support a healthy body and improve your chances of recovery.

Skin and anti-ageing

If you want to become a picture of health as you get older, then a regular routine of juicing is the way to go. Pampering and nurturing your skin from the inside works much better than expensive anti-ageing creams. These delicious tasting juices will slow down the physiological changes that happen as you age. Because juices hydrate the body, your skin will look vibrant and plump. You can easily increase your fluid intake with these delicious drinks and a well-hydrated body is essential for good skin and improved vitality. Before long, people will want to know your secret to ageing so well. If you want skin that glows, get juicing.

Which juicer and blender should you buy?

A big question is which juicer to buy. There are basically three types of juicer: centrifugal, masticating and manual.

Centrifugal juicers

These use the power of centrifugal forces to separate the pulp from the juice and are available in most high-street stores. However, this is not a juicer I would recommend as the high revolutions produce a poor-quality juice. They are quite wasteful on produce as they make a lot of wet pulp, which can become very expensive if you are buying organic foods. Also, the spinning fine mesh basket inside the machine is a pain to wash. A machine that is difficult to wash is the major reason why people who start juicing enthusiastically soon pack it in. This is why I always recommend that you buy a good juicer first and don't waste money on poor substitutes. Another point to remember is if you are juicing every day or juicing for a family, these machines can easily burn out and need replacing. Finally, centrifugal juicers won't juice wheatgrass or leafy greens, they tend to get stuck and can jam the machine. So all in all, I believe they are not the ideal solution.

Masticating juicers

Having tried and tested many different machines, I use a twin-gear masticating juicer (see the Resources section for reputable addresses of suppliers). These juicers have two gears that grind the fruit and vegetables slowly and their unique design uses an extremely gentle and efficient process to extract high-quality juice. They are extremely efficient and produce very small amounts of dry pulp, which ensures you get the best possible yield from your produce. The pulp can even be returned to the chute to extract more juice. As they revolve very slowly while grinding, no heat is produced which is another reason you get a superior quality juice.

There are single-gear masticating juicers that are cheaper but, having tried these, they are not as effective as the twin-gear machines in my opinion. Twin-gear masticating juicers are the best juicers you can buy. They are very versatile and will grind nuts, grains wheatgrass and leafy greens. Treat yourself and start with the best juicer, it's an investment in your health and your future.

Manual juicers

These are very affordable, however they are difficult to use and wash. They are not as good at juicing fresh fruits and vegetables as the electric-powered models. Manual juicers are, however, handy if you are travelling because they are lightweight and portable, which means you can make your own fresh juice wherever you go. They can juice wheatgrass and leafy greens and as a result most people tend to buy them just for wheatgrass juicing.

Wheatgrass juice

This juice has a very strong taste for those who are not used to it, but you can flavour it with lemon or ginger to make it more palatable. If you want to increase your energy and build a healthy immune system, wheatgrass will give you large quantities of nutrients. It is a powerful immune booster that is loaded with minerals, and is rich in beta-carotene, chlorophyll, vitamin C and vitamin B-17 (a substance that is thought to destroy cancer cells). It is one of the fastest-selling super foods in the marketplace, despite its strong taste.

Fresh wheatgrass juice is abundant with chlorophyll, which cleans the blood. The molecular structure of haemoglobin and chlorophyll are practically the same, there is only one molecule different – very simply, the central atom in blood is iron, which helps transport oxygen to our cells, and the central atom in chlorophyll is magnesium, which this supports photosynthesis in green plants.

If you have a cat or a dog, you may have noticed that they often eat grass. This is for two reasons: to obtain nutrients or to eliminate stored toxins and purify the liver. Animals seem to have figured out that healing comes from Mother Nature. Unlike animals, humans cannot digest grass, so it must be juiced in order to utilise its storehouse of nutrients. You can often find wheatgrass juice in juice bars, but it's so easy to grow and cheap to juice your own. If you're too busy to grow it, there are plenty of growers who supply mail order packs of this wonderful powerful cleanser (see the Resources section).

What's the difference between juices and smoothies?

Many people think (incorrectly) that there is no difference between juicing and blending. The difference between a juice and a smoothie is that a juice requires very little digestion when compared with a smoothie. Smoothies can take hours to metabolise, especially if you add bananas. Juicing strains away the juice from the pulp which means that the resulting juice is easily absorbed at a cellular level within 15 to 30 minutes, and this reduces the workload on your digestive system.

I always encourage my students to go for juicing rather than smoothies. Smoothies, however, are beneficial and wonderful for fussy eaters as you can disguise all kinds of nutrients, such as essential fats, raw vegetables and probiotics.

Probiotics offer a great number of health benefits but many of the yoghurt drinks on the market are laden with sugars, so don't be tempted to buy those smoothies. The irony is that the advertisers and food companies don't tell us that drinking probiotics with sugar will encourage the growth of bad bacteria. The biggest job of the beneficial bacteria that live in the digestive tract is to limit the growth of putrefactive and pathogenic bacteria. Also as some of these drinks contain very small amounts of only one strain of friendly bacteria they are poor value for money. Smoothies don't have to include dairy products they can be made with coconut, rice, oat or almond milk. It's so easy to make your own!

Key points to remember

- Make your own, there is no comparison between the freshness of a home-made juice and store-bought juice. Home-made juices will give you a new lease of life and at least you will know what ingredients were used.

- Invest in a good juicer and don't waste money on cheap ones. Cheap juicers are difficult to wash, wasteful on produce and won't juice some of the foods you need.

- Lemon peel can be juiced, but if you are consuming it make sure the lemon is organic to avoid pesticides. The rind of watermelons can also be juiced as they contain beneficial nutrients. Peel produce if it's not organic.

- Use the bruised portions, as they contain salvestrols, a plant equivalent of vitamins that protects our cells.

- Use the seeds of apples, they are loaded with nitrosilides which can help protect us from disease.

- Keep it simple and enjoy. Bottoms up!

7

Shedding those extra pounds

'In the Middle Ages, they had guillotines, stretch racks,
whips and chains. Nowadays, we have a much more effective
torture device called the bathroom scale.'

STEPHEN PHILLIPS

Have you ever been seduced by the latest, greatest diet in your quest to lose weight? So many of my students have been on one diet after another for years with few positive results. They lose weight quickly and then gain it all back, plus some more – they are at a loss to know why their attempts have never worked. They feel it's an impossible challenge and that diets only serve to make them feel deprived and hard done by when they deny themselves the foods they really want to eat. In my experience deprivation never works.

Yet, many people are drawn towards the latest fad diet like magnets, in the hope that this will be the diet that will help them shed those extra pounds. The disappointment they experience when they fail to see lasting results is deflating to say the least.

They are soon tempted by high-calorie, less-than-nutritious food and, before they know it, they reach for whatever snack is in sight. This is a common scenario, one that may even be familiar to you.

But could diets really help you shed those extra pounds? The diets we invest so much time and energy into are not always what they are cracked up to be. Let's call a spade a spade – some of them are a nightmare. Apart from the fact that bingeing and dieting is not good for your spirits, I'm very sceptical of diets because they usually promote some kind of fad or specific way of eating that is unrealistic, unsustainable and not practical in the long-term. If you don't eat proteins, carbohydrates and fats, you are going to have cravings because these are the foods that fuel your body. You need a balanced amount of these fuels for energy, and to help your body grow and repair itself.

Over the past twenty years, selected food groups have been demonised while others have been promoted as health foods. I remember a phase in the early nineties where we were all being told to 'carb-load' – today carbs are the enemy and everybody is into GI diets, most people could even give you the glycaemic load indicator for every food. It's also interesting to see the various food pyramids that are circulated, they vary considerably, depending on current thinking. Then, there was the '0% fat' phase where we all opted for tasteless substitutes. Protein is the health media's current 'in' thing, for as long as that lasts!

What we don't seem to understand is that it is not about any single food group is better or worse than any other, it's about the source of that food that makes us healthy and slim (or not).

We need to take in balanced amounts from each food group. For example, we need small amounts of protein, but your body can best utilise proteins from plants, beans, lentils, nuts and seeds, etc. Again with fats, those that are from plants, such as sunflower, sesame, chia and flax seeds, sprouts and avocado, are the most digestible. As for carbohydrates, we assimilate those most easily from plants, sprouted grains and pulses, vegetables, and fruit.

Is there any point in pursuing the various diets with which we are bombarded especially when there is overwhelming evidence that diets do not work? Low-fat diets have become very popular in our society for the past few decades and millions of people have tried to avoid or lower their fat intake and yet, as a society, we are getting fatter.

The Royal College of Physicians in the UK recently reported the staggering statistics that almost a quarter of adults in the UK are classified as obese and that the incidence of overweight children in the UK has doubled over the past twenty years. Children between the ages of two and 15 years are now being classed as obese. A report published in *Midwifery* gave the first official figures on obesity in pregnancy in the UK. Following a national study, it found that 20 per cent of pregnant women were obese. The National Health Service in the UK reports that, in 2008, 1.28 million prescription items were dispensed for the treatment of obesity, a major increase over the previous ten years.

Is it any wonder that an entire industry has been built around weight loss? The facts remain clear that 'helping' people to lose weight has become big business, and people spend vast amounts of time and money trying to fathom the simple rules of weight loss. Up to one third of men and women in the Western world battle with dieting, and now our children are doing the same. However, overeating is not just a problem for those who are obese. Today, most people in the West overeat.

The good news is that dieting becomes a thing of the past when you move to a healthier way of eating. This I discovered quite by accident when I changed my lifestyle.

Why are we getting fat?

Some experts say that we are becoming fatter because of the reduction in physical activity and they may be right when you consider the fact that we don't even move to change the television channel these days. Others say that our eating habits are genetic or inherited. There are people who live on rich fatty foods, sugary cereals and desserts and develop a selection of lifestyle-related diseases (including heart disease, cancer, arthritis and type 2 diabetes), but who attribute these diseases to genetic factors rather than lifestyle – yet in most cases we get sick from lifestyle-related diseases. I myself suspect it's the increase in consumption of sugars, low-fat foods and fast food that is causing the increase in some diseases that society is faced with.

Are the low-fat, no-fat diets we live on escalating the problem? One thing which is certain is that these foods are definitely not the solution.

Another issue, today, is the huge media attention paid to the dietary habits of celebrities and models. We are constantly evaluating their diets, whether it's the grapefruit diet, the cabbage-soup diet or counting-fat-grams diet. These low-fat diets are bad news for those who decide to follow them as they end up being deficient in essential fats. Good fats are one of the most neglected foods in our diet and this is mostly because of the trends towards low-fat diets. Naturally if you think fats are going to make you fat, you will try to avoid them.

Do you know the difference between good fats and bad fats?

Most people don't really understand the difference between good fats and bad fats. Even the word 'fat' makes us assume that fats make us fat, but that is not always the case. Let me emphasise this point as clearly as I can – good fats do *not* make you fat, *excessive carbohydrates* make you fat. If you restrict your carbohydrate intake to what you burn daily, you will not gain weight.

The misunderstanding about good fats and bad fats has led the majority of the population to try to avoid all fats, but good fats are necessary for health. They keep us slim, help with weight management and they can also improve a sluggish metabolism. Good fats noticeably increase our metabolic rate and energy levels and these, in turn, help us to burn more calories. They increase energy production by helping the body obtain more oxygen and when we have increased energy levels, we feel much more active – and this means we are less likely to crave sugar or carbohydrates to deal with energy dips.

Removing good fats from your diet can, in fact, make it difficult for your body to lose weight. Ironically, if we avoid good fats, we get fatter because we need fat to burn off excess fat. All this nutritional confusion usually leads back to addictive comfort foods. We must remember that small amounts of fats are an intrinsic part of a healthy body – it is not only our figures that suffer from abstaining from these foods but also our health. Good fats are also beneficial for keeping your hair shiny, your nails strong and your skin young looking and blemish free.

Which are the 'good' fats?

One of the best strategies you can employ if you feel you are overweight is to put more nourishing foods back into your diet. There are two essential fats (essential fatty acids) that the body cannot produce and must be obtained from foods. Both are essential for health: omega-3 alpha-linolenic acid (ALA) and omega-6 linoleic acid (LA).

It is important that we get the correct ratio of both fats. We need to add more omega-3 than omega-6 into our diet. People often consume flax oil because it's cheap, but it's only rich in omega-3 and too much omega-3 can lead to omega-6 deficiency symptoms.

Below are some other sources of omega-3 and omega-6 essential fatty acids:

- oils made from sunflower, flax and sesame seeds
- chia seeds
- almond oil
- avocados
- olives

- almonds, Brazil nuts, hazelnuts, walnuts, pecans, pine nuts, pistachios and macadamia nuts (but not peanuts!) – nuts should be raw
- nut butters (but not peanut butter or cashew butter).

Don't let the high fat content of nuts put you off, most of the fat is unsaturated 'good' fat.

To heat or not to heat, that is the question

I never recommend heating fats, such as frying, deep-fat frying and sautéing, whatever method you use it is definitely not good for your health. Subjecting foods to this destructive practice can cause a hardening of the arteries and make blood platelets sticky – and, yes, that includes the good-quality, cold-pressed or virgin oils. Don't use the processed sunflower cooking oils you can get from supermarkets as these oils are easily destroyed by light, heat and oxygen. To make sure you buy the freshest oils, buy unprocessed or cold-pressed oils that have been kept refrigerated and in dark-glass bottles. These oils can be used for salad dressing or added to smoothies, mashed potatoes and vegetables.

Modern technologies have found new methods of processing that enable manufacturers to produce cheap, low-quality oils with a longer shelf life. Good fats are easily damaged and products that contain good fats have a much shorter shelf life. When we heat fats, either by processing or cooking, we upset their delicate balance. The heating process alters their molecular structures and turns them into trans-fatty acids – and trans-fats create free radicals (destructive molecular fragments that are formed during metabolism) in the form of short-chain fatty acids. Oils prepared in this damaging way are better known as hydrogenated or partially hydrogenated oils. You should bear in mind that food manufacturers remove fat from their products to ensure a longer shelf life. Obviously, the longer a product can remain on the shelf, the more profit for the producer and retailer.

Take olive oil, for example. We spend more money to buy extra virgin olive oil which is cold-pressed and unprocessed and is therefore unspoiled. Then we heat it, which makes no sense. When we heat olive oil, it reacts with oxygen and when rapid oxidation occurs, it increases the dangers to our health from the heated molecules. This damages the oil which, as a result, has none of the naturally occurring phytosterols that pure unprocessed olive oil would naturally have. Phytosterols have tremendous health benefits. They help lower cholesterol as they block the absorption of cholesterol from the food you eat, all of which protects us against heart disease. Heated oils are more shelf stable at room temperatures, which for commercial reasons is far more profitable.

Because fats make foods tasty, manufacturers have to add something to the foods to replace the fat that they take out to ensure the food will appeal to consumer's taste buds. I am sure you can guess exactly what they add to improve the flavour – sugar, of course. As you will read in Chapter 9, which is all about sugar, extra sugar or sugar derivatives trigger the secretion of insulin which is our fat storage hormone. Unfortunately, the consumer then experiences cravings, weight gain and low-energy levels. Do they lose weight? Most definitely not!

Good fats stave off that hungry feeling!

Have you ever eaten a meal and soon afterwards felt hungry? Do you scour the fridge for something to eat even though you may have just eaten a large meal? Eating fat-free and low-fat foods gives you that empty feeling. This may be one reason why so many people feel the need for desserts and coffees after their meals. Low-fat foods makes you feel miserable because they rob you of the very foods you need to nourish a healthy body and maintain energy levels.

Healthy fats bring satiety to your meals by giving you the feeling of having had enough to eat. When you have that full feeling, you don't crave sugars and carbohydrates. The body uses carbohydrates for energy, but some are digested so quickly that you soon feel empty after eating them – in contrast when you eat food that contains good fats, you fill up faster and with less food.

A benefit to eating more raw foods is that you need to chew the food and so you don't eat as quickly. Chewing your food sends signals to the brain that you have had enough to eat. When you eat cooked food, you may finish it more quickly and therefore have a 'missing' feeling. Remember that food takes 20 minutes to reach your stomach so you may not feel full immediately after eating. One reason why people overeat is that they no longer recognise the 'full' signal that their bodies send them. It is important to tune into your body's signals at mealtimes.

Imagine, if you can control your hunger, you can reduce your calorie intake. Controlling hunger pangs is an area that food producers have become very interested in. It has become the new diet trend for fighting the battle of the bulge. Food producers know only too well if they can generate sufficient momentum for a fad to take off, people will jump onto the bandwagon and their profits will begin to soar. The future trend to grab people's attention might well be foods that are labelled 'get that full feeling'.

By the way, if you are feeling hungry, try drinking a glass of water or some veggie juice. Thirst is often confused with hunger because our thirst signal is so weak. After you have had a drink wait ten minutes and then decide if you are really hungry.

Portion control is another way to maintain a healthy weight. I have heard so many people blame their spouse, mother or whoever serves dinner for their overeating. I can understand that argument for children, although they rarely use it. You will notice that it is almost impossible to get a young child to eat more than they want, but we lose this inner wisdom as we age. Choose a plate size that will only accommodate the amount you want to eat. Gently explain to whoever dishes out the meals what you are trying to achieve, or serve yourself.

Sit at the table to eat your meals each day. Surveys have shown that when people eat in front of the television, they eat up to 50 per cent more food than they do when they are at a table where there are no distractions.

The benefits

What are the benefits of 'good fats'? Well, they are almost too numerous to list. Below are some of the reasons you should add good fats to your diet. Among other things, they:

- give you energy
- suppress appetite and cravings
- reduce the symptoms of PMT and menopause
- aid the absorption of vitamins and nutrients
- improve brain function and relieve brain fog
- elevate mood and lift depression
- improve heart health by reducing triglycerides
- decrease the amount of plaque in our arteries
- help lower blood pressure
- reduce the risk of blood clots
- reduce inflammation in the body of rheumatoid arthritis
- help lungs, eyes, organs, nerves and cells to function better
- relieve restless leg syndrome
- alleviate ADD (Attention Deficit Disorder) and improve learning
- improve memory
- increase sperm formation.

The list could go on and on.

I hope this list has convinced you how important good fats are for correct functioning of your health. Good fats have the ability to keep us slim and healthy. Don't underestimate them.

You can, of course, try to drop a dress size in two weeks, but most people find that drastic, and find that radical changes don't work for long. It is baby steps not giant leaps that stop people putting the weight back on. If you are to succeed in achieving a healthy weight, it must become a lifestyle change, not something you do for a few weeks and then drop. If you want to be healthier, happier and thinner don't exclude the good fats from your diet.

Key points to remember

- Add more nourishing foods to your meals – the more nourished you are the fewer cravings you will have.

- If you are feeling hungry, drink a glass of water or vegetable juice. Thirst is often confused with hunger.

- Be a bit more discerning of the latest fad that catches your attention.

- Buy oils that are refrigerated and packed in dark-coloured bottles. This stops the oil being exposed to light, which will damage it.

- Eliminate the cheap polyunsaturated vegetable oils, margarine, all partially hydrogenated oils and any foods that contain trans-fats from your diet.

- Stay away from low-fat foods. They often have lots of extra sugar and make you feel miserable because they rob you of the essential fats you need to survive.

- Low-carb foods are also bad news. You need small amounts of carbohydrates to give you energy.

- Be careful of night-time snacking. Snacking in front of the television can pile on the pounds.

- Carbohydrates should be eaten early in the day so they can be used to supply energy rather than being stored as fat.

- Remember that it is not just the food group category (fats/carbohydrates/protein) that is important. Ideally, your food should be from a plant-based, and therefore usable, format for your body to gain nourishment from it.

- Include good fats in your diet. Essential fats are an intrinsic part of a healthy body.

- Celebrate your new found energy. Who knows, it could be the shape of things to come.

8

Weaning yourself off sugar

'If you don't like something change it; if you can't change it, change the way you think about it.'

MARY ENGELBREIT

If you have a sweet tooth, you may even believe that you were born with it or that you won't be able to change no matter what you do. However, it might be time to make sense of why you are addicted to the sweet pleasures of sugar – it may have more to do with your emotions than a sugar addiction.

Sugar addiction stems much further than the physiological needs for sugar. There are a number of psychological factors that contribute to sweet cravings, such as emotions, boredom, moods and stress. We associate eating sugary foods with feeling good and often use sugar as a way of suppressing emotional problems.

If you are worried, bored, stressed or feeling low, sugar makes you feel better and gives that much-needed sense of satisfaction. It can numb painful feelings, ease mood swings, stop us feeling lonely or simply help us pass the time when we are bored. It can fill the emotional void that is left behind from upsets in our lives. It is a lot harder not to reach for the 'quick fix' if you struggle emotionally. If you frequently find yourself reaching for something sweet to relieve unwanted emotional states, then sugar has become your emotional crutch.

When you are stressed bored, lonely, tired, angry or sad, you don't make a salad – you usually reach for chocolate, ice-cream, biscuits or cakes to overcome these emotions. Then you exercise for half an hour as a punishment for your guilty pleasure. If you burn 200 calories what will happen to the extra 400 you have just eaten? Yes you guessed right, its gets stored as fat.

Limiting your sugar intake will not solve all your problems, but it will solve a host of other problems, like managing your weight and blood-sugar irregularities, as well as the disappointment and frustration you feel when you give in to cravings. If you are wary of trying to give up sugar because of previous broken commitments, why not join the growing number of people who have eliminated sugar products from their diets altogether with my help. I'm not suggesting you won't miss it, but learning how sugar affects you can reduce your susceptibility to those sweet pleasures.

Sugar affects your brain chemistry, so don't for a moment think its lack of willpower or self-control that has you reaching for the biscuits or chocolate. Sugar cravings have a lot to do with the brain chemistry of pleasure and reward. Sugar activates the brain to release dopamine, which gives a euphoric effect. That may not sound so bad, but these distortions in your brain chemistry affect your mood and temperament. The temporary high of dopamine that sugar produces soon fades and signals are sent to the brain that triggers more cravings. The more you eat, the less you feel satisfied and, like any substance, it becomes addictive. Changing your body chemistry by changing your diet and lifestyle will help you wean yourself off sugar.

People often tell me they don't eat sugar. What they really mean is they don't eat white table sugar. Sugar is the one food that most people eat every day whether they know it or not, as it is in almost every food you eat. It's no secret that there are hidden sugars in a vast number of commonly eaten foods, ranging from fruit juices, probiotic drinks, sauces, salad dressings, cheese spreads and pretty much every processed food – even infant formula. Those that surprised me most are the ones that are added to savoury foods. Check out the labels of packets of rashers, ham, sliced turkey breast, etc. Remember that anything in an ingredient list that ends in 'ose' is sugar, e.g. glucose, fructose and dextrose.

Today, we are eating more sugar than any other generation. On average, previous generations consumed four to seven pounds of sugar per person, per year. In our modern diet, we eat 90 pounds of refined sugars per person, per year.

Is sugar really all that bad for your health?

Natural sugars have always been present in the human diet. However, previous generations consumed much smaller quantities of natural sugars, found in grains, fruits and vegetables, and these were absorbed along with fibre and other nutrients. When natural sugars are absorbed slowly, it normalises any negative effects of glycemic loading on the body. In other words, glucose enters the bloodstream at a much slower rate when you are digesting complex sugars.

Refined sugars, on the other hand, require little digestion. When you eat refined sugars, you get an instant spike in your blood's glucose level. Refined sugars are like a time bomb ticking within our systems, because our pancreas must secrete large amounts of insulin to stop our blood-sugar levels from rising too high. Every time you eat refined sugary foods, they cause an imbalance in your body chemistry. The extra insulin pushes your system into overload, which tends to make your blood-sugar levels fall to levels that are too low. The type of energy we obtain from refined sugars is short-lived and causes a fast rise in blood-sugar levels that may then lead to an adrenaline surge. This is usually followed by an abrupt slump – so the relentless cycle starts again.

This constant yo-yoing between high and low blood-sugar levels means your unfortunate body is faced with the challenge of trying to restore balance. These extreme spikes in blood-sugar levels and constant insulin demands, mean that your pancreas cannot respond and cells begin to shut down. The result is that you end up tired and lacking in energy.

Yet, despite all of this, we delude ourselves into thinking that we need just a little something sweet to keep our blood sugars stable. Of course this is nonsense, because far from maintaining blood-sugar levels, your system is pushed into overload by keeping your blood sugars on a constant roller-coaster of highs and lows. Once you begin to balance your blood sugars, you will start thinking logically and rationally about you sugar fix.

Cholesterol is another problem caused by sugar derivatives, such as high-fructose corn syrup which is in hundreds of foods. High-fructose corn syrup can increase LDL cholesterol (bad cholesterol), which is a risk factor for cardiovascular disease. Even salad dressings are often laced with large amounts of high-fructose corn syrup. The more sugars that are added to your food, the more of it you will eat. Food companies count on you developing an addictive relationship with these foods.

Cancer cells thrive on sugar. They have many more receptor cells for capturing sugar than healthy cells. The molecular biology of cancer cells requires glucose to feed them. For some people, cancer cells grow faster and stronger when their sugar levels are frequently above normal. Cutting down our intake of sugar cuts off an important food supply to cancer cells. It's not just people who are diagnosed with cancer who are affected by this. Each of us generates new cancer cells each day in our bodies – but a healthy immune system deals with them so that they don't become an issue.

It's clear that we need to take a serious look at overcoming the tendency we have to consume too much sugar, when research shows that sugar:

- increases your risk of cancer and diabetes
- elevates LDL cholesterol
- disturbs brain chemistry
- increases weight and obesity
- raises blood-sugar levels
- increases the risk factor for kidney disease

- feeds fungus, yeasts and bacteria
- rots teeth.

Health may not be an overriding factor when it comes to the melt-in-the-mouth pleasures of sugar but, as research has shown, there are consequences to the foods we put into our mouths each day. However, no matter how much we hear about the dangers of eating sugar and sugar derivatives, its sweet temptation is such that we ignore the devastating effects it has on our health, which is why we go back again and again for more and more. Since sugar and chocolate are synonymous with pleasure, does it really matter that there are a range of problems associated with it? Sugar's mouth-watering pleasures have a strong hold on us. You may not want to admit this at first because the idea of going without a treat is not easy.

While these habits are not always controlled by rational thinking, they can be changed. Easier said than done, you might say – and at one stage these were my sentiments too.

The prospect of the sugar blues may seem daunting and I understand that you may not want to give it up completely. Most of us manage it for a week or two, but eventually we slip back into having 'just a little treat' and then we are hooked once more. But as I have said, habits can be changed. Once you get to grips with your sugar addiction, you will reap substantial health benefits as your blood sugars become more balanced, you drop excess weight and save your teeth from rotting.

How to reduce sugar cravings

Let's look at some practical steps you can take to help you break free of this addictive substance. If you are going to fight off the urge for the momentary pleasures of sugar, you need to develop some tactics to help improve your chances of succeeding long term. Remember it takes some time to create these habits, so it's going to take time to undo them.

To reduce the intensity of the sugar cravings that occur when you start going without your sugar fix, take some chlorella supplements. Chlorella is an inexpensive source of pure green algae, which helps reduce sugar cravings and will keep you from unnecessary snacking. It helps balance blood-sugars levels, which is essential if you are to succeed in getting rid of your sweet tooth.

Chlorella is also rich in chlorophyll which helps purify the blood. If you suffer with constipation, it cleans out the bowels, cleanses the liver and removes toxins which is advantageous to those who drink alcohol or smoke. It encourages tissue repair, absorbs carbon dioxide and releases oxygen, which is necessary to support a strong immune system. It is also beneficial to people who need rebuilding after an illness. It's rich in protein, omega-3 fatty acids and macronutrients. Make sure you purchase chlorella that has had the outer cell wall broken down, the tough cell walls of this form of algae can slow down digestion and absorption of the product. Also check with your doctor before taking chlorella if you are on blood-thinning medication.

One of my readers recently wrote on my Facebook page:

After a couple of weeks of a sugar fest, I am back on mega helpings of chlorella. I haven't had any choccy cravings so far. I think that giving up sugar might be like quitting cigarettes for me – one slice of chocolate gateau and I'm climbing the walls for more. I have a spare bottle of chlorella in my handbag at all times. Thanks for letting me know, it's keeping me on the right track.

Find a healthy replacement to your usual treat. When I started down this road, I used to get my sugar-fix from an apple. Originally I had varied the fruit throughout the day but this ended up with me eating a vast array of fruit and so I was taking in sugars of another kind – fructose. When I kept it to one simple fruit, I only ate it to solve the craving, not to indulge my taste buds, and that kept me from overdoing it. In time, I was eating only a modest few apples a week and now I no longer use them as a crutch.

If this isn't enough for you to overcome the brief pleasure of sugar, why not allow yourself a weekend treat in the initial stages just to get you over the hump. Now that doesn't seem so bad after all, does it? But, here's the deal, you must make sure you have to leave home to get it. Hopefully by now your cupboards and freezer are cleansed of those guilty pleasures.

You may think a weekend treat will only perpetuate the problem, but it stops you feeling hard done by going without your fix. Mums often used this tactic with kids when they are trying to limit their sugar intake so see if you can manage to do the same. I usually encourage people to avoid, rather than resist temptation, because I strongly believe if you don't buy sugary foods, you won't be tempted to eat them. However we have to be realistic at the outset as I know only too well that sometimes the spirit can be willing, but the flesh can be weak. This is a compromise during the transition stage.

One thing I have learned while teaching is how people respond to incentives. Responding to incentives may be as innate as any other instinctive human behaviour. Looking forward to a reward motivates you into going the extra mile. The weekend treat will help to train your mind to adjust and will help you to become less dependent on your sugar treats. The secret is to make it a treat – not a habit.

We cultivate a sugar addiction in our children. For most of you there is no need to specifically outline the dangers and downsides of sugar for our children in particular. You may have been victims of mood swings, hyperactivity, tantrums and attention deficits. We cannot blame the children when we have taught them that sugar is a reward for good behaviour, it's a celebration food or an indulgent treat.

You could try giving gold stars on a chart – it seems to work for super nanny! My own favourite for the smaller ones is balloons or bubbles as treats, colouring books or comics as they get older, and nothing cuts it like cash with the teenagers! I know it's more expensive that a party pack of jellies but it will change the atmosphere in your home for the better once the sugars are gone.

Healthy substitutes

Find healthy substitutes for those sugar cravings. Try some of my new recipes, it's so easy to make delicious nutritious treats from almonds, raisins and coconut. Natural plant sweeteners like stevia are good replacements for refined sugars. Stevia is about 4oo times sweeter than sugar, a half teaspoon of stevia is equal to one cup of sugar. It has been used in Japan for years to replace sugar, where over 300,000 pounds of stevia is consumed each year. Stevia actually helps to regulate blood-sugar levels and has become widely available as a sweetener since its approval for use by the EU in 2011. It comes in liquid and powder form, I recommend you use the liquid version as the powered version does not dissolve well in liquids. Don't surrender to the melt-in-the-mouth products any more, there are really good alternatives out there.

Cinnamon is also a great blood-sugar regulator. Sprinkle it over cereals or into warm drinks or take a supplement to help overcome the sugar-demons.

Be on your guard with artificial sweeteners

There are many artificial sweeteners which people use as alternatives to sugar. Not only are some of these toxic but some of them can actually stimulate your appetite and increase your cravings for sugar, which is all bad news for your waistline. Almost a quarter of additional calories come from added sugars. Know the truth about artificial sweeteners. Ignorance is most certainly not bliss in this case. Here are a few to watch out for:

- Aspartame is a well-known sweetener that has been linked to many diseases. According to research, this controversial non-nutritive sweetener can cause heart palpitations, breathing difficulties, anxiety attacks, tinnitus, vertigo, memory loss and joint pain. It is found in cereals, flavoured water, cooking sauces, yoghurt, diet soda, chewing gum and even children's medicine.

- Saccharin is used in restaurants as a replacement for table sugar, it's also used in soft drinks, chewing gum, jams and baked goods. Saccharin was previously listed as a cancer-causing substance by the National Toxicology Program in America. Saccharin was banned, as recently as 2001 in parts of America, but is now been deemed safe, however, I would err on the side of caution with this artificial sweetener (see www.epa.gov). People chew sugar-free gum to protect their teeth and enhance their breath, check if your gum contains artificial sweeteners.

- Xylitol is a white substance that looks very like sugar. It is a sugar alcohol that can be extracted from plant materials. Xylitol is marketed as a 'sugar-free' sweetener and is often used in place of sugar because it has fewer calories and reduces the risk of tooth decay. Nonetheless, it can cause diarrhoea and raise blood-sugar levels.

- High-fructose corn syrup is derived from corn which may seem harmless enough, but it can raise blood sugar as it consists of 55 per cent fructose and 45 per cent glucose sugar. There has been an increase in the use of this sweetener by manufacturers because foods maintain a longer shelf life with this additive, and it is inexpensive. It's found in breads, soft drinks, ice-cream, ketchup, salad dressings and a host of other common foods. You may think that diet drinks have fewer calories, but research suggests that drinking diet soda can stimulate fat storage.

Whether you are focused on your waistline or your health, reducing or eliminating as much sugar as possible from your diet, regardless of what type it is – is most definitely the way to go. Even raw honey, although natural, is high in fructose, and though this has health benefits, it should be used in moderation as it is absorbed as a sugar in the body. Agave syrup is another natural sweetener often advertised as a natural sugar. Remarkably, many health advocates recommend agave syrup or agave nectar as a healthy alternative to sugar. They don't inform you that it's processed, high in fructose and causes unwanted weight gain. I used it myself in the early years until I learned it is just another sugar. Others to watch for are cane juice, dextrose, lactose, glucose, maltose, fructose and malt syrup.

Naturally, if you are a self-confessed chocoholic, you're going to crave something sweet. In order to resist temptation, why not attach some negative thoughts to your favourite treats? Every time you fancy a bar of chocolate, biscuit or a dessert, tell yourself it's destroying your teeth, putting on extra weight and raising your cholesterol levels. If sugar is strong enough to penetrate through tooth enamel, can you imagine the damage it can cause within the body?

Motivating yourself with daily affirmations of the health benefits of eliminating sugar can help you trade in your sweet cravings for a more discerning palate. Okay, you may be sceptical about how this could help you break your sugar addiction, but if you allow yourself to be free from judgement and to be open to new approaches, you can make the choice to change the negative patterns of behaviour you have been stuck in over the years. Only when you make a conscious and deliberate effort to look at your behavioural tendencies can you strip away the negative belief habits and behavioural patterns that have become entrenched over the years.

Adding a negative association to sugar can change the way you think about it, and this is well recognised as a useful mental tool to help those wishing to kick harmful habits like smoking. Developing feelings of revulsion towards the foods you are compelled towards can be a simple yet very effective way of giving up those foods. For example, if you imagine your favourite treat tasting like a food you hate. When you see your sugar habit from this perspective, it soon begins to lose its attraction. We all get stuck in old habits but, by doing this, you will stand a much better chance of fighting off the urge for sugar and overcoming cravings.

Finding out the dangers associated with eating sugar can be hard to take on board. Giving up sugar for me was the culmination of many steps. If you are to make a consistent change in curbing your sugar cravings, it has to come from within. We all blow hot and cold when transitioning away from unhealthy lifestyle choices. If you cannot alter your thinking, you may perpetuate the very situation you need to change.

Key points to remember

- Clean your cupboards and refrigerator of anything you know will tempt you. Don't make it harder than it has to be. It's much easier to avoid, rather than resist temptation.

- Try making some healthy alternatives, there are lots of recipes to entice you in the treat section in Chapter 17 (see page 237). Their sweet taste will trick your body into believing you have eaten sugar.

- Chlorella supplements are also useful in helping you get over your craving, as they regulate blood sugars.

- If you must, allow yourself a weekend treat. It helps you cut down gradually, and you are less likely to end up overindulging farther down the road.

- Be prepared for those cravings. Stock up on nuts and seeds, you can buy spicy or garlic nuts that taste delicious. Keep them at hand in your car or desk drawer, they are a perfect snack if you are on the road. Nuts and seeds are packed with protein and are a good source of vitamin E, magnesium and riboflavin. They have a low-glycemic number and will curb hunger almost instantly.

- Use stevia, a natural plant sweetener, to replace refined sugars. Stevia has a low glycemic load which means it won't raise your blood sugars.

- Stay away from artificial sweeteners as they may cause more sugar cravings and stimulate your appetite.

- Adding a negative association to sugar can change the way you think about it. It's a useful mental tool to help you kick those harmful habits.

- Get plenty of rest, stabilising your blood sugars overnight is important. If you are deprived of sleep, your body finds it difficult to control blood sugar.

- Don't let your belly rule your mind.

9

Living without dairy

'No matter what you believe, it doesn't change the facts.'

AL KERSHA

Do you believe that milk is wholesome and builds strong bones? You may be startled to know that, contrary to what most of us believe, cow's milk is not the perfect health food to build strong bones in humans. We assume that milk forms strong bones because advertisements tell us so, but did you know that advertisements claiming that milk builds strong bones have been banned? The myth and hype that has been built around insufficient calcium intake is strongly linked to marketing and advertising.

Food processing companies clearly use our concerns for health to promote and sell their products. If they can connect their products to our concerns that we will not get sufficient calcium or proteins, they are onto a winner. The ease with which distorted information is spread through advertising proves how easily we accept these practices. Huge monetary rewards can be gained by generating sufficient interest in the foods available in shops.

The core of the dairy lobbyists' argument is that we will not get enough calcium to sustain strong bones if we don't consume 'enough' dairy products when, in reality, consuming dairy may actually lead to poorer bone integrity in the long term. Studies show that calcium robs minerals from bones, which weakens and subjects them to arthritis and osteoporosis. The Harvard School of Public Health (see www.hsph.harvard.edu) states:

> Studies suggest that high calcium intake doesn't actually appear to lower a person's risk for osteoporosis.

Harvard researchers also reported that 'there was absolutely no link between milk consumption and bone density'.

Dr Neal Barnard, the Head of the Physicians' Committee for Responsible Medicine, based in Washington DC, has said:

> It would be hard to imagine a worse vehicle for delivering calcium to the human body … While scientists are hard at work searching for specific breast cancer-fighting compounds, the safest approach is to apply what we already know: [Eating] diets that are highest in a variety of plant foods and stay away from heavy oils, meat, and dairy products, helps prevent a great many diseases. The earlier in life we start, the better.

Food companies don't highlight the fact that milk has the ability to influence our health in a negative way. They fail to address adequately the fact that cows are exposed to pesticides, antibiotics and eat grass that has been treated with chemical fertilisers.

Intensive farming is another issue. Cows are forcibly impregnated yearly and are milked while they are pregnant, which is a time when these animals have increased levels of oestrogens. Do you really want another animal's hormones in your system? The unfortunate animals are forced to produce about four and a half times more milk than they naturally would to feed their offspring. A normal healthy cow produces about four to five litres of milk each day, whereas working dairy cows produces on average 25 litres of milk a day.

Epidemiological research suggests a correlation between milk consumption and at least two kinds of cancer – especially the hormone-related ones, breast and prostate. It's well-publicised that Oriental women consume few or no dairy products and have very low rates of breast cancer, while it has reached epidemic proportions in many Western countries. Is there some lifestyle factor that is seriously increasing the Western woman's chance of contracting breast cancer?

Dr Colin Campbell's *China Study* points out that the growth factors that are contained in dairy products increase insulin-like growth factor-I (IGF-I), which is an aggressive promoter of cancer and abnormal cell growth. Are dairy products a significant dietary component that has contributed to the staggering increase in breast cancer cases amongst Western women? The evidence is pretty compelling when we address the fact that the Chinese also have the lowest rates of osteoporosis in the world and yet consumed few or no dairy products.

Campbell's alarming research shows that casein compounds are a chemical carcinogen and have been found to be a deadly cause of cancer. Caseins are a group of proteins found in cow's milk and they constitute about 87 per cent of the total proteins in milk sold.

Through his 25-year study into animal proteins, Dr Colin Campbell has contributed to public understanding of the potential health hazards of drinking dairy milk. Campbell states:

> We could turn on or turn off cancer growth by increasing or decreasing the amount of casein. Lesions that normally remain dormant, with a steady dose of cancer promoters in the diet may override natural defences against the growth of tumours.

After years of scientific research, he continues to work tirelessly to expose the risks of drinking milk.

Caseins also encourage the formation of mucus, especially in the gastro-intestinal tract. Basically, the human body does not require milk after weaning because, by that stage, we produce less of the lactase enzymes necessary for its digestion. Lactose is made from one molecule of glucose and one molecule of galactose. It is a disaccharide, a type of sugar, that must be broken down in the small intestine by lactase enzymes – if it is not properly absorbed, it ferments in the digestive system and is the cause of many digestive problems.

Initially these problems may be identified as digestive upsets and diarrhoea but, eventually, they cause inflammation in the mucous membranes and lungs. The sticky mucus produced by consuming dairy products needs to be excluded for a variety of reasons, but mainly because of its effects on the arteries – it will stick to your tubes like glue. This outpouring of mucous causes ear infections, a runny nose and persistent sore throats – all of which are recognised as some of the clear allergic reactions that are accentuated and triggered by dairy products. A high percentage of the world's population is unable to digest the milk sugar, lactose. These people cannot drink cow's milk because they get allergic reactions, known as lactose intolerance – milk literally makes them ill.

I can honestly say that I have noticed an enormous difference since I gave up eating and drinking dairy products. I no longer suffer from congestion in my chest if I get a cold. Asthma, blocked sinuses, ear infections and allergies can all be alleviated by cutting out dairy. Most of us recognise if we have a negative response to specific foods, so it is important to go with your instincts in these cases.

Emma, the wife of a dairy farmer, wrote to me recently:

> When Jack was born, I wanted to give him the best start and so struggled through the difficult first stages of breast-feeding. He cried a lot and we realised that something wasn't right. His tummy was distended and he got severe rashes for no reason. People tried to be helpful and they all had their own theories such as 'some babies just cry a lot' or 'he just has colic'.
>
> At five weeks old, I had him tested and we discovered that he was intolerant to foods he had access to through my breast milk. When I avoided these, he improved considerably. Even though dairy was not listed as a problem food, I was acutely aware of the affects it was having on him. Any time I ate dairy products, Jack became snuffly and congested, and when I had a hot milky drink, the symptoms were even more distressing. Every mum becomes tuned in to the various

sounds of her baby's cries and I knew that my son's system was having a bad reaction to dairy products, in particular milk, ice-cream and cheese.

Removing dairy from our diet was not a decision that I took lightly due to the fact that I am married to a dairy farmer. However, I feel very strongly about doing what's best for my son. My husband too has seen first hand some of the negative effects of dairy foods.

I am now much more aware of the affects different foods can have, especially the negative effects. The added bonus for me was that my own sinus problems have disappeared and my skin looks better than ever, and we have each had one cold in the past year and a half. I now want to eat foods that offer us both positive benefits and nourishment, to give Jack the best start in life, and so that I am fit and healthy to enjoy him for many years to come.

This young mother recognised not only that dairy milk was having an adverse effect on her but that she was passing those ill effects on to her baby through her breast milk.

Butter, cream and cheese products have the same downsides as milk, and they are also high in cholesterol and saturated fats. High cholesterol, hardening of the arteries, heart disease and stroke are caused by saturated fats.

Even when these products receive bad press, food companies conduct their own studies in the hope of countering any allegations that are put forward. Their opinion cannot really be described as impartial and when the results are triumphantly produced after frenzied attempts to justify the value of their products, consumers feel relieved that their familiar food is after all not damaging to their health and they go back to using it. Objective achieved for the food company.

Most people are victims of the advertising that they have absorbed like sponges throughout their lives.

If you think you don't consume a lot of dairy products check exactly how much you are taking in – the obvious ones are cheese, yoghurt, probiotic drinks, cream and butter. But, like sugar, milk is hidden in a lot of foods.

Some cereals, cereal bars, crisps, processed foods, deli meats products, frozen desserts, and bakery and confectionary products contain casein, non-fat milk powder or whey protein. It's really important to check for milk-based ingredients, especially if you are lactose intolerant.

Where will you get calcium if you don't eat dairy?

For many people, a big question is: If I don't eat dairy, where will I get calcium? Let's be clear and give a straightforward answer to this question: It is *not* a lack of dairy that gives you brittle bones and decreases bone density it is a lack of weight-bearing exercise. Strength training strengthens the joints and bones, not consuming dairy products. Today, we lead more sedentary lives, we sit in front of computers and televisions, and often only engage in small amounts of physical activity.

Preventing bone loss is about more than calcium intake. Bones are like muscles, and they need to be worked in order to say strong and healthy. Any physical activity which causes muscles to contract will help lay down more bone and improve bone density. Carrying shopping, gardening, push-ups, dancing, skipping, lifting weights, swimming and yoga are all good ways to help your body maintain strong healthy bones. As the saying goes, use it or lose it.

If you can't bear the thought of lunges, squats or lifting weights, try a vibrating plate machine. The technology was developed for astronauts after their long, weightless trips in space. Bone and muscle loss is a major problem for astronauts as their bones can weaken alarmingly when they do not have the limitation of gravity. This type of exercise equipment tones muscles and increases bone density. You stand on the vibrating platform and carry out a series of exercises in order to develop strength and muscle tone. It is a fast and effective way to stay in shape. I find it helps me stay in shape without having to spend hours in the gym. These machines will set you back a bit as they are quite expensive unless you are a member of a gym that has one. Otherwise lunges, lifting weights and squats can be done with minimal expense.

Large mammals, such as elephants and silverback gorillas, have huge muscle structures and do not suffer from brittle bones or osteoporosis and yet, they eat *no* dairy foods. These animals get all the calcium they need from the raw vegetation they live on. Of course, cow's milk contains calcium, but this calcium was meant to be consumed by baby calves, not humans. Humans cannot digest the calcium obtained from cow's milk, in fact this type of calcium bonds with other calciums in your body to accelerate calcium loss.

Understanding which foods have absorbable calcium is important because there is no point taking in calcium if your body cannot absorb it. Vegetables have far more absorbable calcium than dairy milk. Not only is the calcium better assimilated by the body, vegetables also have significant amounts of other nutrients that improve bone health.

Is milk as healthy as you think!

Do you believe it's wise to drink the milk of another species? Nature does not intend the milk produced by one species to be consumed by another creature. For example, dogs don't drink milk from cats, or horses from cows but, then again, animals are wise enough to use their instincts. Although domesticated cats drink dairy milk, this is more because of conditioning by humans.

The thing that should strike you about our habit of drinking milk is that we are drinking a white liquid secreted from the mammary glands of an animal that uses it to feed its offspring.

Think about that for a moment, if you saw a lactating animal secrete a white liquid would you drink it? What makes it more acceptable when we get it from a carton in the supermarket? Why don't we drink milk from a horse, a cat or a dog?

Humans have not evolved to drink milk from another animal. There are major differences in the composition of cow's milk and human milk. Human breast milk has the correct levels of protein, carbohydrates, fats, vitamins and minerals to feed a growing baby. Cow's milk is meant to support a rapidly growing calf to develop to a half ton weight in less than two years. Cow's milk has more proteins and digesting these proteins places an enormous strain on the human digestive system – cows have four stomachs; humans have one. Also humans do not need milk after weaning, in fact we are the only mammals that continue to drink milk after weaning.

Because milk formulas for infants have been criticised as poor substitutes for mother's milk, Chinese scientists have been working on a genetically modified herd of cows to find a substitute for mother's milk. Researchers at the Chinese Agricultural University introduced human DNA into dairy cow embryos and they have created cows that produce milk similar to the profile of human breast milk. Writing in *PLoS ONE*, Professor Li Ning, the project's leader says:

> As our daily food, cow's milk provides us the basic source of nutrition. But the digestion and absorption problems made it not the perfect food for human beings. The genetically modified cow's milk is 80 per cent the same as human breast milk.

Who knows what might happen to the children of the future if they begin to drink genetically modified milk.

Your basic beliefs about milk being a healthy nutritious food might be shattered when you learn that milk contains alarming amounts of pus. Yes, that's right, pus (or somatic cells as they are routinely called). Milking machines suck so hard on cows udders that they get wounds and infections. Cows get mastitis, which is a bacterial infection on the teat which means the cow must then be treated with antibiotics. Mastitis is like an abscess that is full of accumulated pus. This produces high levels of somatic cells (white blood cells) in milk. A somatic cell count is used to measure the quality of milk.

Milk that is approved for human consumption meets permissible somatic-cell-count levels, which really means that milk can be sold which contains permissible levels of pus and blood. In Europe, the generally accepted (EU milk quality standard) of somatic cells is 400 million (pus cells) per litre. This is not a distorted statement about our milk supply – it is fact. One teaspoon of milk could contain up to 1 million pus particles.

Despite the rules regarding the cleanliness of commercial milking equipment and stringent testing that milk goes through, there is still a risk of pus residues and hormones getting into the milk supply.

Dr Robert Kradjian, Head of the Chief Division of Breast Surgery at Seton Medical Centre, wrote an open letter to his patients, advising them about milk. In it he said:

> Any lactating mammal excretes toxins through her milk. This includes antibiotics, pesticides, chemicals and hormones. Also, all cows' milk contains blood! … the USDA allows milk to contain from one to one and a half million white blood cells per milliliter. Another way to describe white cells where they don't belong would be to call them pus cells.

So, let's ask: Will pasteurisation eradicate all the bad stuff?

You might think that because milk is pasteurised, the heating process will kill off bacteria but, if this is the case, why is it necessary to have accepted levels of pus cells in milk? Also various components of milk, such as fats, are altered by the heating process. One of the destructive effects of homogenisation is that heating fats turns them into fermented fats which are carcinogens (cancer-causing substances).

For various reasons, we are more accustomed to sweeping these things under the rug. It's obvious that there is a real need to change our views and misguided beliefs about consuming dairy products.

You may be sceptical that a food that generations of people have consumed could be harmful to your health. Maybe after reading this chapter, you might change your perception of milk. Whatever you decide make sure your decision is not controlled by vested interests.

I certainly came to the conclusion that dairy products are not the perfect health food that I had been led to believe they were. What I found lacking was scientific support for consuming foods that have adverse effects on the body. As you can imagine, there is much controversy about the value of dairy foods but there *are* problems associated with this food source and its production.

Key points to remember

- Substitute cow's milk with good replacements, such as unsweetened rice, oat or almond milk.
- Eat or juice more dark-green leafy vegetables as they are rich sources of calcium and are an economical and absorbable way of increasing your calcium intake.

- Sesame seeds, have almost 1,000 milligrams of calcium per 100 gram serving. Sprout the seeds to make their calcium more digestible.

- The humble wholegrain quinoa not only possesses good amounts of calcium, it's also rich in proteins, potassium and zinc. Quinoa can be sprouted and added to soups just before serving, so its nutrients are not destroyed during the cooking process.

- To encourage greater calcium absorption, take a food grade vitamin D supplement each day. Vitamin D is crucial for the absorption of calcium. I recommend supplements that are only made from foods such as shitake mushrooms or algae (contact b@changesimply.com).

- Expose your skin to 20 minutes of sunshine in the early part of the day to obtain adequate amounts of vitamin D. If you are unable to get adequate sun exposure, you must take a supplement.

- For bone health, limit foods that slowly deplete calcium, such as sodium.

- Reduce your consumption of carbonated soft drinks. Soft drinks contain phosphoric acid which accelerates bone loss.

- When you exercise try weight-bearing and muscle-strengthening exercises to build bone density. A fast and easy way to build bone is to use a vibrating plate machine. The vibrations tone muscle and increase bone density.

- Remember humans do not need to consume milk after weaning.

10

Putting some spice in your life

'We are indeed much more than what we eat, but what we eat can nevertheless help us to be much more than what we are.'

ADELLE DAVIS

Spices have been traditionally used for their therapeutic properties.

Turmeric

The turmeric root is a valued condiment that adds flavour and a pronounced yellow colour to food. Indian physicians have always used turmeric, or *haldi* as it is known in India, to treat arthritis, dysentery and ulcers. But it is not just the Indian people who have recognised the wisdom and complexity of this amazing natural spice. Millions of Indonesians, Japanese and Chinese people are also familiar with the powerful healing properties of this natural root. Even in the West, the potent plant compounds in turmeric are considered to be the most powerful healing rhizome (the underground stem of the plant) on the planet.

In recent times, turmeric has received a lot of publicity because of its anti-cancer effects. Statistics show if you take 1 million women in the USA, 660 of them will develop breast cancer and 160 of them will not survive. If you compare that with 1 million women in India only 79 will develop the disease and only 41 will die from it. For prostate cancer in men, the statistics are just as dramatic.

Turmeric is part of the curcuminoid family of spices. Curcuminoids have been scientifically shown to enhance brain function and directly inhibit the enzymatic activity of COX-2, an enzyme that helps regulate inflammation and pain. The curcumin element in turmeric prevents the enzyme from even forming.

The therapeutic, medicinal properties of curcuminoids have not gone unnoticed by the pharmaceutical industry. The biological activity of turmeric as a healing agent explains why companies are interested in it and why they have filed for so many patents. The curcuminoids group of natural compounds can be easily isolated and synthesised which makes them suitable for drug formulations.

The Indian government successfully overturned a patent application for turmeric. In 1993, a patent was filed by the University of Mississippi Medical Centre in America for the use of turmeric powder as a wound-healing agent and the patent was granted in 1995. The New Delhi-based Council of Scientific and Industrial Research challenged the patent, and the US patent office upheld the objections, which lead to the subsequent cancellation of the patent. Dr R. A. Mashelkar, an

Indian scientist, alerted the Indian government to these issues. A spokesman for the government said:

> We will not allow anyone to patent something that we have known about for thousands of years.

Turmeric can also be taken in supplement form which is useful if you are not making spicy food each day. The supplement delivers high concentrations of this natural wonder. Watch out for supplements that contain synthesised additives to ensure you are not ingesting chemical solvents. It takes about two or three months before you get the full benefits of this herbal remedy. If you are pregnant, check with your medical practitioner or naturopath if you can take supplements.

Turmeric and arthritis

In addition to its anti-cancer properties, this pungent deep-yellow powder is also useful for healing wounds, aiding digestion, relieving pain and reducing inflammation. Since inflammation is responsible for playing a large role in many diseases, if you have arthritis, rheumatism, muscular problems or memory loss, you should add turmeric to your daily diet and ensure you are getting good quantities of it.

This potent natural anti-inflammatory has no adverse side-effects unlike many anti-inflammatory drugs available on prescription. Clinical trials from Italian researchers reported that patients were able to decrease their medication of non-steroidal, anti-inflammatory drugs by 63 per cent. The researchers reported a dramatic drop in pain and stiffness and increased flexibility in their patients who use the turmeric formulations.

At the other end of the spectrum, researchers at Columbia University Medical Center provided data that showed the most commonly used bone-building drugs (bisphosphonates) may actually lead to poorer bone density in the long term. They found there was a noted suppression of bone restoration that lead to brittle bones when these drugs were used for four or more years.

At low doses, there are usually no contraindications between the turmeric root and pharmaceutical medications, but you need to check with your medical practitioner or naturopath for their advice. My husband used large amounts of the supplement to help relieve his painful arthritis. The turmeric did not cause any complications, unlike the drugs he was prescribed when he was first diagnosed with the condition. Although he is not exactly a follower of natural remedies, he will not miss his daily dose of turmeric. When he is away from home or on holidays and forgets to take it, he finds that the pain and stiffness returns.

Cumin

Cumin seeds have a nutty, peppery taste and they are a key ingredient of curry powder. The seed can be bought whole or ground into a powder. It is rich in iron, which is a vital component of haemoglobin. Cumin is also rich in calcium, manganese and magnesium. It slows down free-radical damage in the body and research show it has anti-cancer effects.

I like to add cumin to crackers and curry (see recipes on page 221). This culinary spice gives a good kick to crackers, soups and sauces. I use the seed rather than cumin powder, as the seeds can be easily ground with a mortar and pestle and they don't lose their flavour as quickly as the powder.

Ginger

This is another excellent anti-inflammatory root and rhizome. I absolutely love adding it to my green juice. It gives it a lovely warm taste, especially in the winter months when drinking cold juices can seem unappealing. Ginger is very effective in treating morning sickness as it blocks a neurotransmitter that can trigger nausea.

I well remember how my mother used to give me a warm ginger drink for a queasy stomach. She never read a health book in her life, yet she instinctively knew what foods helped each specific ailment. Just like turmeric, ginger takes a while before you get its full effects. It's also very effective at preventing colds.

Cayenne

Cayenne is another amazing spice that is useful for the heart. Cayenne pepper improves circulation and it help to clean and maintain the cardiovascular system. It has a variety of other therapeutic properties that has earned it its healing reputation. It calms ulcers, lowers blood pressure and it is used to coagulate blood from cuts and wounds. For cuts, apply ground cayenne powder directly to the affected area and cover with a bandage. Be warned it will sting but it does a fantastic job. The virtue of this natural product is it provides effective, long-term relief.

Cayenne can be added to a glass of water first thing in the morning to improve circulation. It also adds a nice kick to bland meals. It's extremely hot, so use it very sparingly until you get used to its peppery taste. I use it on nearly everything instead of pepper. Try it in hummus, soups, curries, crackers and sauces to give them extra flavour. I don't know how I ate food without it.

Cinnamon

Cinnamon has many medicinal uses. For example, it can help decrease blood-sugar levels, it is believed to improve digestion and it is used for colds, nausea, diarrhoea and painful menstrual cramps. Cinnamon can also reduce LDL cholesterol and some compounds in cinnamon can thin the blood. The rolled cinnamon sticks can be grated into warm drinks or the ground powder can be sprinkled over cereals or oatmeal as an alternative to sugar.

**

The old saying 'variety is the spice of life' has always been true, and with health-care costs on the rise, it might be well worth taking a closer look at the benefits of these medicinal plants and spices.

If you are looking for more natural remedies, try these healing spices. They are cheap and they have no side-effects. As consumers learn more about their health benefits, I have no doubt they will find that putting some spice into their life will be a valuable addition to a healthy diet.

Key points to remember

- Use turmeric for its anti-cancer and anti-inflammatory properties. If you don't want to add it to your food, it can be taken in supplement form as the supplement delivers high concentrations of this amazing spice (contact b@changesimply.com).

- Cayenne is useful for the heart. Add it to water first thing in the morning to improve circulation and to help clean up the arteries of the heart.

- Cumin's nutty, peppery taste adds a nice flavor to crackers, breads, soups and sauces and, of course, curries.

- Ginger can be added to your juices and it gives the juice a lovely warm taste. Ginger is very effective in treating nausea or a queasy stomach and colds.

11

Ditching the coffee

'Success seems to be connected with action. Successful people keep moving. They make mistakes, but they don't quit.'

CONRAD HILTON

Have you ever toyed with the idea of giving up your favourite brew? If you are a coffee drinker, it's all too easy to become dependent on your daily hit of caffeine. Working long hours in stressful conditions and consistent decision-making can lead you to reach for that much needed cuppa. There is no doubt that it gives you a lift. However, that temporary increase in energy you experience is short-lived and, before you know it, you're having three or four cups a day just to keep yourself ticking over. A love affair with coffee can easily spiral. You enter a relentless cycle of addiction and craving, it can happen with sugar too. As you become more addicted, you begin to build up a tolerance for caffeine and it takes more and more coffee to get that original hit.

Coffee has it highs, but it also has its downsides. It can make you feel irritable, lethargic and can give you headaches. Caffeine raises levels of the stress hormones adrenalin and cortisol and, similar to blood-sugar swings, your body struggles to adjust to increased levels of stress hormones in your blood. When we are consistently pumping adrenalin, it keeps the body in a 'fight or flight' mode (the response when danger threatens). People who exist on adrenalin don't know how to slow down. Looming deadlines and working under high-pressure conditions seem to be a normal part of modern life. Not only are these lifestyles difficult to sustain, they are also addictive. As the pace of life becomes more and more frantic, a stressful lifestyle is often the reason people rely on stimulants to help them get through the day. These busy and pressured lifestyles are far more demanding than we realise and they pose a very real health risk.

If you are trying to kick the coffee habit, it might be worth identifying what causes you stress and seeing if there are ways you can reduce your stress levels. Stress is notorious at driving you to reach for a comforting quick fix. Don't just soldier on and suffer in silence, it's important that you understand the emotional reasons behind your need for stimulating drinks. Getting out of the rut will help you start to eliminate stress from your life.

Even if you have tried your best to stop, there is more you can do. Make it your business to find out why you reach for these types of addictive substances. Is it because you are stretched in all directions? Is it because you get a sugar hit? Is it to keep you awake? Is it the social aspect? Is it just a habit? Once you identify the reason, you can eliminate it. You have to get back to the root of the problem if you are to figure out its cause.

Stress

If the reason you drink coffee is stress look at what is producing stress in your life. Are you putting everybody else's needs first? Are you failing to say no when you should? Are you ignoring your own physical and emotional needs?

Money problems are one of today's most common stressors and can be a constant worry. It is so common to dwell on the things in our lives that are not going well and our propensity to worry penetrates into the mind. Worrying is not good for anyone's health. Whichever situation is responsible for producing tension in your life – money, work, family – it needs to be consciously looked at with a view towards altering it.

You might say that it's only a few cups of coffee, but if you are drinking coffee to alleviate stress, then the solution to giving up coffee is to learn how to fix your stress problem. Coffee will contribute to the problem as it plays a part in making you feel tired, restless and irritable. It does this by suppressing serotonin, a neurotransmitter that prevents tension and depression.

If you are sitting in front of a computer screen all day, chances are the reason you are drinking three or four cups of coffee each day is to keep alert. Technological progress has contributed to our stress levels. As technology slowly gains ground in our lives, it brings a new level of anxiety with it. The question is: Are you a net-frazzled fanatic addicted to surfing the net, social networking, checking e-mails and text messages? While your conscious mind may not recognise these things as being stressful, your body feels the effects of habitual distractions of constant communication.

Internet addictions contribute directly to stress problems and sleep disturbances. So-called 'bloggers' addiction' has been known to keep people up all night.

Once you've identified if this situation applies to you, you can decide to shut out the volume and strain of the overload of information and get some extra rest. Getting to the root cause is the best way to successfully restore some balance to your busy life. It's well worth working on these aspects of your life. Once you've taken action – any action – you don't feel so powerless.

The social aspect

Lots of people drink coffee because it's part and parcel of their social lives – think of all the times people say, 'Let's meet up for coffee.' Sharing a cup of coffee with a friend and having a nice chitchat keeps the social sphere going. Sharing time with friends not only elevates your mood but it can create a general feeling of wellbeing.

There is nothing like the smell of freshly ground coffee to make you want to hang out in a cafe. I fully understand how easy it is to get caught up in drinking lattes, mocha-chinos, long blacks or double shots of dark roast.

I no longer drink coffee but I can remember visiting a friend in Portugal before I quit. She was a bit of a coffee connoisseur who liked a strong cup of dark coffee – and she drank one on the hour, every hour. It didn't take long before I gave into the pressures of joining in with the Portuguese way of living. Portuguese life is punctuated by the pleasures of coffee drinking and there are an incredible number of coffeehouses there.

It was considered rude not to drink the local brew. Out of politeness to my hostess, I downed several strong espressos each day, it seemed the right thing to do at the time. Despite the fleeting high that I got, after a few days of drinking coffee continuously, my head was pounding. I was awake during the night and I began to feel the need for another shot. I was even on the brink of using something to help me sleep!

I was so wrapped up in all the socialising and holiday spirit that I barely noticed how much coffee I was drinking. I reckon if I had stayed with her for much longer, I would have become a certified junkie. Fortunately, I managed to tone down my zeal for coffee when I returned home, but I must say I still love the aroma of freshly ground coffee beans.

I know some people who managed to quit their much-loved four or five cups of java by going cold turkey. Then again, there were others who quit and ended up drinking a lot of diet sodas. Swapping one bad habit for another is not the answer. Maybe it's a testament to the power that caffeine has over people.

James was a participant on one of my courses who liked his coffee. He wrote to me after the course:

> For the record, I found your course very uplifting and helpful, though I still struggle to stay firmly on track all of the time. I've fallen off the wagon a few times, but now I'm very aware that I'm doing so … the perennial problem of sabotaging

oneself, against inner knowledge baffles me. However, on the plus side, I no longer take coffee. That's now a definite no-no that I'm finding easy to maintain even though I was a severe coffee addict.

James made progress in other ways too, he gave up dairy and he started sprouting and growing wheatgrass, which is a great result for a beginner. Well done, James!

You have probably noticed that people are starting to drink coffee at a younger age. In fact, according to the statistics, teenagers are now the fastest-growing sector of coffee drinkers. Why this is the case I am not sure. It could be late nights, cramming for exams or the social aspect. I suspect one of the reasons is that coffee shops are safe places for teenagers to hang out. But raised levels of stress hormones in teenagers brought about by caffeine may not be such a good idea. It may only be a matter of time before pent-up aggression and mood swings set in, and these are sure signs of caffeine addiction. Professor of Neuroscience at John Hopkins University, Roland Griffiths has stated:

> Caffeine is likely the world's most-used, mood-altering drug and it does produce mood changes and physical dependence and withdrawal. It needs to be recognised as a drug.

Weight loss

Whether you want to give up coffee to cut calories or to eliminate caffeine, there are many benefits to quitting coffee. On the bright side, you may be cutting back on a lot of milk and sugar which will definitely be good for your figure and your health.

Losing weight is a very good incentive to encourage you to quit, particularly if you eat while you drink. More often than not, people consume biscuits and cakes whilst they drink coffee. Decreasing the amount of sugar and those indulgent sweet treats reduces the calorie disadvantage of those three or four drinks. Remember all that sugar adds up. Sweeten with stevia to reduce your sugar intake. Stevia comes from a plant and has a low glycaemic load so it won't spike your blood sugars. This should be a priority if you want to lose weight.

Drinking coffee is regarded as a possible cause for the build-up of cellulite on your body. Cellulite is misshapen fat. Coffee can cause a build-up of chemicals and toxins that cause cellulite to form under the skin. Caffeine can also promote the excretion of calcium which is yet another good reason to ditch the coffee habit.

Take a break

Part of the attraction of coffee drinking is taking a break. We develop a soothing attachment to our morning or afternoon breaks. It provides a nice opportunity to help your brain chill out. Having a warm drink can create a shift in brain activity which can help clear the mind. A simple tea break can help you relax, unwind and escape from all that multitasking.

Many people also drink coffee out of boredom. It's a pick-me-up that has a certain high. It relieves the humdrum tedium of domesticity and work. It can be an interruption between tasks or a reason to take a break from your work. However, try to make it the exception rather than the norm as small subtle changes can make a difference.

Another incentive is the money you could save on all those lattes, espressos and frothy cappuccinos, which has to be good. If you tot up how much you spend each week on your coffee-to-go, you might be surprised.

Giving up

If you love coffee and cannot bear to be without the taste and aroma of your creamy, foamy cappuccino sprinkled with chocolate, then there is probably no point in me trying to convince you to give it up totally.

But you should try. Find a substitute to get you through those first few weeks. There are a few really good caffeine-free coffees. They come in different flavours – java, almond, amaretto – and really taste good. You will find them in good health-food shops or on the internet.

Although coffee drinking is on the rise, tea is the second-most consumed beverage in the world after water. What could be more relaxing than to stop and sit for a few moments and savour the soothing flavour of a simple brew? It is a wonderful antidote to our noisy and busy lives, but try switching to herbal teas, they are especially refreshing and calming.

Herbal teas are rich in antioxidants, which are beneficial for health and wellbeing, and they will help to get you over the longing for coffee. You can source herbal teas that will give you a lift and refresh you. Green tea, for example, will still give you a slight caffeine hit, but not as much as coffee. Rooibos tea is another fantastic pick-me-up. It's high in antioxidants, vitamins and minerals, and has no caffeine. Interestingly, Rooibos is sometimes given to babies for colic.

There are other teas that have a calming effect and induce relaxation almost immediately such as Valerian, which is a well-known herbal sedative. It brings about a sensation of calm, especially if you suffer from insomnia or if you are restless and your mind is racing so you can't sleep. Camomile will help you unwind at the end of a busy day. This one is very good for people who suffer with nervous tension or mild anxiety and it's great before bedtime.

Peppermint is my favourite. It reduces bloating and helps relieve indigestion by increasing the secretion of digestive enzymes. I like to sit in my garden with a nice cup of tea and smell the mint leaves. It gives me a few minutes to soak up the atmosphere. Changing your immediate environment can change your perspective on stressful issues and events. You move into a different mindset when you connect with nature.

Lemon and ginger are fantastic on a cold winter's day. Ginger aids digestion, I grate the fresh ginger and just add some lemon. You get more flavour from freshly grated ginger than from a teabag. Nettle tea is super for cleaning your blood system as it is rich in chlorophyll. It is also high in silica, which is great for skin and hair.

Start with fruit teas if you need a sweet taste, but gradually move to the herb teas which are much more beneficial. You will be spoiled for choice.

There are some other great positives to ditching the coffee habit – your concentration will improve and you will sleep soundly when you manage to kick the habit.

Ultimately, less is more – less coffee leads to a more vibrant you.

Key points to remember

- If you feel like you are drinking too much coffee, try to reduce it by one cup per day to begin with. This will reduce your caffeine dependency and bring you one step closer to quitting.

- If you are finding it hard to resist, distract yourself by eating an apple. It will start the process of eating for health rather than comfort.

- Try caffeine-free substitutes that are made from grains. While they are not the real thing, they will help you adjust to living without your daily hits of caffeine.

- Make sure you drink lots of water. Coffee is a diuretic that causes your body to eliminate water which has a very dehydrating effect on the body.

- Switch to herbal teas. Green tea will give you a slight caffeine hit and ease the withdrawal symptoms of caffeine.

- Sweeten with a few drops of liquid stevia to reduce your sugar intake. This is great for your figure and you will soon get used to its taste.

- If you feel exhausted and stressed, take some down-time. If that's easier said than done, perhaps you need some stress management.

- Curtail unnecessary internet use during your time out and get some extra rest.

- Most of all, celebrate your successes. Best of luck!

12

Eating out

'You only live once but, if you do it right, once is enough.'

MAE WEST

Eating out is something we all enjoy. It's wonderful to share a meal with family and friends but whether it's a holiday, an event or a night on the town, staying healthy in a social situation can be a bit of a challenge. Eating out is a time when most people let their guard down, it's a time when we allow ourselves to indulge, let go and enjoy ourselves.

While I've always loved eating out with friends, I've realised that this is not the healthiest pastime. It's hard to decide what to do if everyone else is stuffing themselves with food and booze, especially if they expect you to do the same. Today, this seems to be the cultural norm and although you may be with friends, you may still feel awkward or intimidated. The comforting familiarity of your old habits may be more socially acceptable to friends or family.

If your friends are a party-hard crowd, they might feel you are judging their less-than-perfect habits if you don't join in. If they feel threatened or guilty, you may begin to experience their disapproval. I have seen this problem time and time again, I am afraid it's human nature to stifle the enthusiasm and efforts of others when we don't want to take part. If your family and friends are giving you a hard time about changing your eating habits don't be discouraged, remember it's a learning curve for them too. Who knows, they might eventually come round to your way of thinking.

Social acceptance is important to the majority of us and the desire to fit in is something that most of us can relate to. You don't want to risk social ostracism, so you give in to keep the status quo. Then you have to contend with that nagging voice at the back of your mind that tells you that you have undone all the good work you've put in so far, and that you should have gone for the healthy option on the menu.

Trust me when I tell you that there are ways you can look after your health while mixing with friends.

My advice is not to preach, as this could end up in an argument, which will taint everyone's enjoyment of the evening. People don't like to have their comfort zone disrupted and they can become intimidated if you become a goody-two-shoes holding forth about the benefits of your healthy choices. It's a wonderful gift to share your experience with others and to see the positive effects it has on their lives, however I normally steer clear of preaching the benefits of lifestyle changes to those who are not up for it.

I completely identify with the fact that you might be eager to share your experience or feel compelled to pass on to others what you have learned. During the early days of finding out this information for myself, I wanted to tell everyone what I had learned so they too could improve their health, but I soon learned that people are impervious to change, not everyone is ready for it. At this stage, I understand that they have little tolerance for these subjects if they have no interest in them.

Family and friends have a huge influence on our lives but think about it, what is the best part of socialising? It's connecting, catching up and having a laugh. Well I am wholeheartedly up for that, and I am lucky to have a great network of friends and family, most of whom are light-hearted and fun. Having a good laugh is an instant, natural mood elevator that releases endorphins (health-enhancing hormones) and creates more serotonin, a neurotransmitter that helps combat stress. As the saying goes, laughter is the best medicine.

The common bonds we share with family and friends are both enjoyable and important because they fill our lives with meaning and purpose. At a restaurant, focus on conversations and catching up, rather than the food and drink, and soon those close to you will accept your choices when they find your still fun to be with. You will find after a while they won't even notice your 'eating habits'.

When you become more health conscious, you meet others who have the same interests and healthy eating becomes the norm when you start socialising with this group. Mixing with other health-conscious people can also prove to be the best possible way forward for you if your family and friends are not really accepting of your new regime. Unless you have support, you could find yourself derailed.

Ask for what you want

Yes, of course it's harder to stay on track when you are out of routine, but you do not have to cancel out all the previous weeks' effort to stay healthy and in shape in one night. If you think changing your lifestyle means your days of eating out are over, the good news is that most restaurants these days offer more healthy options. Finding delicious food is easy if you ask, so don't be shy. I find most restaurants are very accommodating and will create a meal to your liking if you let them know of your preferences at the outset.

Recently we were out for a meal with some friends and although it was a good restaurant, the healthy options were pretty poor. I found nothing on the menu that I fancied so I spoke to the waiter and he was more than happy to oblige with something special. The chef enjoyed showing off his talents and when the food arrived the others commented on how tasty it looked. I was pleasantly surprised and the food was absolutely delicious.

Paying more attention to your health makes complete sense, so don't be afraid to ask for what you want. If you are too embarrassed to ask for something to be made specifically for you, you can always say you are allergic to certain foods and you will find that restaurants will definitely be more accommodating. Asking for what you want encourages restaurants to add healthy foods to their menus. One of my friends who travels internationally and does a lot of entertaining has an e-mail he forwards to restaurants and hotels when he is making a reservation. He finds this works really well as they are informed of his exact requirements and it means he does not have to spend time explaining in front of his guests when he arrives at the restaurant. In case a spontaneous dinner crops up, he also carries a small card with his food requirements printed on it for the waiter to give to the chef, which is a great idea.

Not every restaurant you go to is guaranteed to provide a range of healthy meals, so think ahead and book restaurants where you can have a choice of tasty and healthy dishes. When possible, go to restaurants you know and trust. Try dining in Indian, Thai, Chinese and Middle Eastern restaurants, as they usually cater for vegetarians and vegans and have the greatest choice of these types of dishes. Even fast-food restaurants have become much more health conscious and now offer garden salads and baked potatoes.

Concentrate only on the foods that you can eat, rather the foods you can't. The 'can have' list of foods leaves less room for poorer choices. Positive focus on what to add rather than what to deprive is the key to success. You will soon begin to notice and enjoy the benefits of this simple tactic.

Learn to say no

The downfall of most people is the yearning for something sweet to finish off a meal. We've all been there – now you need to learn how to handle this new situation. If you don't want to have that slice of chocolate gateaux or that slice of tempting cheesecake don't be coaxed into it. Be prepared for the moment when the desire for life's sweet pleasures overrides all the progress you have made. There will be the moment when you say, '*I'll start again tomorrow.*'

If you have made significant progress in weaning yourself off sugar, eating a dessert might well spark cravings and you will be hooked once more. To get through those difficult moments, remember why you made changes in the first place. Look on the bright side and think about the payoffs – weight lost, more energy, clearer skin, fewer PMT/menopause symptoms and last, but not least, better health. Don't be pressured into eating or drinking things you don't want to. I have a friend who heads for the ladies to touch up her make-up when the desserts arrive, she finds it stops the temptation. If you are still having your weekend treat save it for the evening you are socialising. Now you're still in with the gang but you have not backtracked on your plan.

If you are going to a friend's house for dinner and you're concerned that they may not have a healthy option for you, have a small snack beforehand to take the edge off your hunger. I always offer to bring a hearty salad with me – at least then I know that I'll have something wholesome and tasty. When you start eating more healthily, your salads seem to become more interesting than they used to be and you will find that others will be delighted to share them. Opt to be the designated driver, it has its advantages – you don't over indulge and you don't end up with a hangover in the morning.

The recipes in Chapter 17 will help you establish better eating habits and give you options for making your lifestyle changes work long-term, without feeling deprived or socially isolated. There's not a lot more to say about eating out, except enjoy and have fun.

Key points to remember

- Offer to book the restaurant so that you know it is somewhere that you have interesting and healthy alternatives. Check out the restaurant menus online don't forget that there are entire websites that accommodate this such as www.menupages.ie.

- Have (dairy-free) soup or a salad as a starter. Just because it's a salad it does not mean it has to be boring. Ask for hummus, tapenade, pesto, nuts, seeds or beans to add texture and interest.

- Salads, vegetable stews, curries and baked or roast veggie dishes make good main courses that are filling and satisfying.

- Avoid dishes that are fried, as oils become carcinogenic when they are heated. Choose instead raw veggies, and baked, grilled or steamed dishes.

- Ask what is in the sauce or gravy. If you're unsure, ask if they can give it to you on the side.

- Don't preach to friends. Remember they may not be ready for change. They might eventually follow when they see how well you look.

- Learn to say no. If you don't want something don't be pressured or coaxed into eating or drinking it. Stand your ground and decline the offer without fuss.

- On nights out, focus on conversations and catching up with friends and don't emphasise the food element in your mind.

- Concentrate only on the foods that you can eat, rather the foods you can't. That way you won't feel deprived.

- If you deviate occasionally don't beat yourself up. Enjoy the evening and don't feel guilty, but get yourself back on track as soon as possible.

- Most of all, acknowledge and appreciate your results.

13

Spring cleaning your colon

'I wish that being famous helped prevent me from being constipated.'

MARVIN GAYE

Now, I want to get down to the nitty-gritty details of cleaning out your bowels.

Constipation is one of the most common gastrointestinal complaints and one of its main causes is dehydration. Your body's systems depend heavily on water. When you are dehydrated, your body's response is to decrease urine output in order to conserve water. Urine then becomes yellow in colour and more concentrated and may have a strong odour.

Water not only hydrates your body, it also prevents constipation and assists the detoxification process which is essential to maintain good bowel health. Your organs cannot function well without water, so your body prioritises their needs first, compromising the wellbeing of other bodily functions. As your body tries to prevent water loss, it extracts water from other areas: the lymphatic system (which removes toxins from the body), the blood stream (which carries oxygen around the body) and the colon (which removes waste), not to mention your skin and your joints. When water is pulled from the colon, stools become hardened. Impacted faecal matter then begins to accumulate on the wall of the colon and this can contribute to a build-up of toxins. The accumulation of faecal matter in the colon can lead to inflammatory bowel disease and colon cancer.

I cannot tell you the number of people who tell me they only have a bowel movement every week or ten days. Irregular bowel movements can set the stage for future problems with the colon.

If you suffer from a bloated stomach or flatulence, cleaning out your colon will help alleviate these problems. Dr Kellogg, the famous surgeon and the creator of Kellogg's Corn Flakes, believed the colon was the origin of most diseases and he had a point, most of the toxins in the colon come from the foods we eat.

It is so important to have regular bowel movements to remove any backlog of leftover waste from the colon. If the colon is not functioning properly, gas, putrefaction and fermentation arise. Water cleanses the colon naturally and flushes out toxins and waste. It helps produce mucus in the colon which neutralises faecal acids and assists bowel movements to pass more easily. Faeces are usually 75 per cent water, with the remainder being digestive juices, fats, proteins and bacteria.

Cleansing from the inside is every bit as important as cleansing on the outside.

Start your day with two glasses of water and lemon juice. Drinking water is a great way to hydrate and cleanse your body first thing in the morning. This is such a simple tip but nonetheless an important one. Drinking water early in the day helps your body to kick start the cleansing and elimination process. Water is essential for eliminating waste substances and toxins from the colon.

Don't let stomach problems impact on your life. There are many simple ways to get to the bottom of these problems – literally. In order to help your bowels function properly, raise your knees into a squatting position when going to the toilet, the raised angle helps the body eliminate waste fully. You might think this is crazy or cringe at the thought of squatting while going to the toilet, but the conventional sitting position slows elimination and causes wastes that is not fully removed to stick to the colon wall. Squatting is the natural position of elimination that man has used since the beginning of time. Raising your knees when going to the toilet is a great tip for those who suffer with haemorrhoids as it reduces straining during evacuation. You can use a small foot rest to raise your legs into a squatting position, this will ensure an uninterrupted flow during elimination and gravity will do the rest.

As mentioned, the problem is that some people have sluggish bowels or impacted waste on the walls of the colon that has built up day after day, week after week and month after month. This waste gets jammed in between the crevices and villi in the colon and is extremely difficult to eliminate with normal bowel movements.

Villi are small, cellular, finger-like projections that protrude from the lining of the intestinal wall and can trap faecal matter, causing a slow transit time of faecal material through the gut.

'Transit time' refers to the amount of time it takes for waste to leave the colon. A slow transit time causes the waste matter to decay and ferment. The stored waste is a breeding ground for bacteria and the longer the body is exposed to this waste material, the greater the chance of disease. Autopsies have shown that a huge proportion of the population have large amounts of foul-smelling impacted waste in their colons. The colon is the body's sewage system. We would not allow our toilets to back up with waste for a few days much less weeks or months, so why let this happen to our bodies? The best way is to increase your body's transit time is by having regular bowel movements. One bowel movement each day can still leave about three meals' worth of decaying food inside you.

Another problem that can arise is not being able to answer nature's call when you get the urge. For instance, you could be in the middle of a meeting, driving your car or on a bus where it is just not possible for you to go to the toilet. When you postpone a bowel movement, liquid waste gets reabsorbed into your body. It is absorbed into the blood stream and carried through your body's systems. These liquid wastes and poisons increase the risk of infection. So don't put it off for long.

Colonic irrigation

I am often asked if colonics are a good way to eliminate waste from the body. Colonic irrigation is a process where a water-based solution is inserted into the colon through a tube in the rectum to flush out faecal matter. If you have ever had a colonoscopy, your doctor may have recommended this type of colon cleansing in preparation for it. There are, however, pros and cons to this type of intervention.

When the bowel is functioning correctly, it eliminates waste material and bacteria naturally. If the colon is overloaded with waste material, it becomes sluggish and enlarged. If elimination is not complete, it puts pressure on adjacent organs, and the nerves that control the prostate, bladder and uterus become stretched and distorted. An obstructed colon is not effective at expelling newly formed waste because it must pass through a much smaller passage. This is where a colonic irrigation can be useful, as it removes the impacted food material that has built up over time. They are also useful at clearing toxins and parasites that populate the gut.

Apart from ridding the body of unwanted waste, there are other benefits to having a colonic. You may experience some weight loss after a colonic therapy because once the waste material has been removed, the body becomes much more efficient at passing faeces through the unobstructed gut.

Colonics are also a sure-fire way of detoxifying the liver. The liver eliminates toxins and filters poison from the blood and if it becomes overloaded with toxins, your health can be severely compromised. The liver secretes bile for the digestion of food into ducts. If these bile ducts become blocked the bile is prevented from being carried to the intestine and instead accumulates in the blood. Colonic hydrotherapy treatments stimulate the production of bile from the liver and the bile receptors open and release bile into the ducts. The discharged bile is then released and flushed out of the body. This type of cleansing is effective for transporting free radicals and toxins out of the body.

You should be aware that colonic irrigation can initially cause side-effects, such as cramping, bloating and dehydration. I do not recommend long-term use of colonics as they strip the gastro-intestinal tract of not just bad bacteria, but also good bacteria and this increases the risk of infection. If you have a colonic make sure you ask the therapist who is administering it for an implant of wheatgrass or a good probiotic afterwards. It will only take a few minutes extra to administer an implant and it will ensure that you replenish the gut with healthy intestinal bacteria.

Enemas

A gentle way to cleanse the colon is with an enema, which is similar to a colonic insofar as it is a procedure that introduces liquids into the rectum. However, unlike a colonic, an enema only reaches the lower part of the descending colon. The tube is connected through a narrow hose with a nozzle to an enema bag which holds the liquid. When inserted, the lukewarm water or herbal liquid fills the lower intestinal tract, the extra fluid can cause a powerful peristalsis, which is an urgent need to empty the bowels. You may feel uncomfortable or experience some cramping for a short period. A hot-water bottle will help with cramping after taking an enema. Be careful when inserting the tube into the rectum, use coconut oil to lubricate the nozzle and never push if you experience any pain. Cleanliness is important when using enema equipment, so ensure you wash the nozzle of the tube thoroughly after use.

Enemas work faster than laxatives. If you have mild constipation, increasing your water intake and taking some flax seeds will usually sort out the problem, but if you prefer an instant cleanse, enemas are worth a try. Enemas can be carried out in your home at any time throughout the day. A colonic can be used occasionally if you feel you need a deeper cleanse.

Natural colon cleansers

A good cleanse can work wonders.

- Flax seeds soaked or ground into cereals or smoothies first thing in the morning can help enormously if you have a constipation problem. Flax seeds are a good source of insoluble fibre which sweeps faecal matter out of the colon. The seeds help produce bulky thicker stools, which may at first cause uncomfortable bowel movements, but this will soon pass, if you get my meaning.
- Bentonite clay is a simple and natural way to cleanse the colon. This is edible clay that is made from a combination of water and volcanic ash. It acts as a laxative by absorbing water and soaking up poisons, much like a porous sponge. It then forms a gel which takes toxins and waste out of your body. Start out with a teaspoon of clay mixed thoroughly in a large glass of water. After a few days gradually increase the amount of clay you use by a quarter of a teaspoon.
- Psyllium husks are a good source of pure dietary fibre. Like bentonite clay, they act as a sponge in the gut, swelling as they absorb water and faecal matter in the bowels. This produces a soft, bulky stool that assists in a faster passage of waste through

the colon and aids evacuation. Take about a teaspoon an hour before meals. Stir the psyllium husks into a glass of water and drink immediately. Make sure to drink plenty of liquid with each serving.

- Slippery elm is a popular ingredient often used in laxative teas. Slippery elm is a herb from the inner bark of the elm tree. The herbal preparation contains chemicals that may offer some relief from stagnant bowels, as it causes mucous secretions which relieve stomach and intestinal problems. It is available in capsule or powder form and can also be used as topical antiseptic treatment for wounds and skin infections.

Flax seeds, bentonite clay, psyllium husks and slippery elm are all available in good health stores.

Cabbage, celery (in fact most fruit and vegetables), sesame seeds, walnuts, raisins and prunes are also readily available sources of insoluble fibre. Don't forget the important thing is to drink plenty of water to clean excess mucus and congestion out of the colon.

Headaches

Headaches are often triggered by dehydration. Very often we use medications to alleviate symptoms of headaches when, some-times, drinking more water would be enough – though, of course, that does depend on the severity and the frequency of headaches. Frequently, we believe that thirst is the indicator that we need to drink more liquids. But thirst is one of the last signs of dehydration of the body's systems. You lose substantial amounts of fluids through perspiration, urination and bowel movements before you realise that you are thirsty.

Drinking in between meals

It is much better not to drink while eating and digesting food. We are so accustomed to washing down food while eating that it is difficult to break the habit. We enjoy eating and drinking at the same time, but when you drink during meals, you dilute the hydrochloric acid in your stomach, which is needed to break down foods into a liquid state. If your gastric juices are diluted, it can interfere with digestion and lead to acid reflux and heartburn. Try drinking fluids up to a half hour before a meal and one and a half hours after a meal. Drinking away from meal times helps with the absorption of nutrients.

Clean water is indispensable for good health, so drink lots of it.

Key points to remember

- Constipation is often caused by dehydration, so increase your intake of water to relieve this condition.

- Add a teaspoon of flax seeds soaked or ground to cereals or smoothies in the morning.

- Try an enema to cleanse the intestinal tract instantly.

- Answer nature's call. Don't postpone a bowel movement – you don't want waste to be reabsorbed into your blood stream.

- Place your feet on a foot stool when going to the toilet. The raised angle ensures an uninterrupted flow during elimination.

- Don't dilute your gastric juices. Hydrochloric acid needs to be strong in order to break down foods into a liquid state. Therefore, drink between meals, but not immediately before or after eating to aid digestion.

14

What's in your tap water?

'Children of a culture born in a water-rich environment
have never really learned how important water is to us.
We understand it, but we do not respect it.'

WILLIAM ASHWORTH

Some problems associated with tap water have been publicised
in the media, but many of us have little understanding of
the sources of the contamination we are exposed to through
our tap water, which contains measurable amounts of several
contaminants. You may think twice before drinking tap water
when you discover it contains toxic chemicals, such as chlorine,
fluoride, lead and aluminium.

A recent report by the Drinking Water Inspectorate in the
UK revealed that despite widespread purification treatments,
pharmaceutical drugs are finding their way into the water supply.
Another report from the Environmental Protection Agency in
America revealed that in a single year, 2.4 billion pounds of
cancer-causing materials were released into the environment and

stated that much of these cancer-causing toxins and chemicals found their way into water and food supplies.

Most water authorities have based their approach to supplying water on the World Health Organization criteria for what is safe and use disinfectants, such as chlorine and chlorine dioxide, to reduce the health risks from disease-causing pathogens and organisms in source water. However, problems arise when these chemicals react with one another.

Chemical compounds commonly used for disinfection can create new chemical formations, such as trihalomethanes, which are closely associated with cancer. These new chemicals can be toxic when they react with naturally occurring organic matter in water. Their efforts to control disease-causing germs and pathogens, such as e-coli and cryptosporidium, gives water suppliers the consequential problem of having to limit the risks from disinfection by-products. Simple logic dictates that this is not going to lead to better health.

Fluoridation of our water supply is a completely unnecessary practice that has serious health implications for all of us. Fluoride is absorbed through the small intestine into your blood stream and your kidneys must work hard to remove it. The amount that remains is stored in soft tissue, including the pineal gland in the brain, all of which poses a significant risk to your health.

In February 2012, the European Commission warned that the very youngest are at greatest risk, with bottle-fed babies receiving 140 times more fluoride from formula than from breast milk. Many babies are fed formula that has been made up with fluoridated tap water and yet parents have not been warned of the risks.

Fluoride was first added to drinking water in the 1960s because it was thought that it would reduce tooth decay. Even though medical science has progressed since then, it would appear that we in Ireland have not taken notice of the serious health warnings that the vast majority of European countries have acknowledged. This unnecessary medication and crude practice has been totally discredited by 98 per cent of European countries who have condemned and banned this treatment from their water supplies, citing serious medical and ethical concerns.

Contrary to popular belief, fluoride causes dental fluorosis (permanent pitting and discoloration on the enamel of teeth). At least 30 per cent of children exposed to fluoridated water show an increase in dental fluorosis.

When you study the medical literature on the fluoridation of water, there appears to be no logical reason whatsoever for continuing with it. It is an antiquated practice. We must question the ethics of adding a toxic chemical to our drinking water when its long-term health effects are unknown.

Harvard University published a study by the National Institute of Environmental Health Sciences demonstrating how fluoride in water can cause permanent neurological damage to children. The Harvard study, along with 26 other scientific studies, found that fluoride is a dangerous neurotoxin.

This supports the findings noted in the esteemed Professor Joel Kauffman PhD, who concluded in the *Journal of American Physicians and Surgeons*:

> There is evidence that fluoridation increases the incidence of cancer, hip fractures, joint problems, and that by causing fluorosis it damages both teeth and bones. Other medical problems may also occur, including neurological damage. Fluoridation of municipal water should cease. Individuals should remove fluoride from their tap water if fluoridation cannot be stopped.

We sometimes have an unquestioning belief in the old ways of doing things. My belief is that it is we who are suffering as a consequence of this unethical, unnecessary and outdated practice and my recommendation is that you should avoid drinking tap water if at all possible, unless the chemicals are filtered from it.

Is the price of bottled water hard to swallow?

Do you wonder if bottled water is safer to drink than tap water? You may think that bottled water is free of nasty chemicals and toxins but it's a sobering thought to realise that some bottled water is just overpriced tap water. Today, bottled water is big business, we consume billions of litres each year and it is now nearly as expensive as petrol. For some families, bottled water has become a costly addition to the family budget, but is it worth buying bottled water if it is no safer than your tap water?

Think about it, what is it that makes you pay for bottled water? Is it the label that has convinced you that the water comes from a pure spring and is the best-quality water to drink? Or do you just grab the first bottle that comes to hand without question? If you're going to spend your hard-earned cash, you need to know what you are paying for.

Of course, some bottled water comes from pure natural springs and wells, but are you aware that several commercially produced bottled waters can come from public water supplies? Because of clever packaging, consumers might have a false impression that they are buying pure spring water, when really the water is treated tap water that is minimally filtered and sold on to them.

Why are we are so trusting of these manufacturers? Can we honestly believe they have our best interests at heart when we can see plainly that concerns for our health have been grossly obscured by the drive for profit? If only we could cut through the half-truths of clever marketing, it would be more cost-effective for our health. I am all for people drinking more water – I have talked about hydrating and drinking more a lot in this book – but if you drink bottled water, you need to check its source.

Plastic drinking bottles is another area that you need to check out. Plastic bottles that hold water have trace amounts of potentially hazardous substances that are transferred from the plastic into the water. Some of these substances pose a health risk, for example BPA (Bisphenol A) molecules have been associated with heart disease and diabetes. Canada banned plastic baby bottles that contained BPA in 2008. Pthallates are another compound that make their way into water. They come from plastics and agricultural chemicals and mimic the effect of oestrogen on body tissues.

The Goethe University in Frankfurt, Germany, examined the potential exposure to endocrine-disrupting chemicals as a result of drinking water that had been stored in plastic bottles. They declared that these bottles contaminate drinking water with xenoestrogens (foreign oestrogens), contaminants that are invisible to the naked eye. The water may look clear, have no smell and even taste fine, but the fact is that it is not fine. When we drink contaminated water, we burden our immune systems with a toxic load that builds a foundation for disease.

These contaminates have the potential to interfere with oestrogen and other reproductive hormones by tricking your body into thinking that it is processing oestrogen. Xenoestrogens are also known to play a part in the onset and progression of cancer. Remember that store-bought bottled water sits in warehouses or on the shelves for months where it has plenty of opportunity to leach foreign xenoestrogens from the plastic into the water. Sometimes, you may leave your plastic drinking bottles in your car and they sit in the sun where the heat causes toxins from the plastic to seep into the water. I have on many occasions seen pallets of bottled water stacked in yards behind supermarkets, left sweating out in the elements with no apparent realisation of the damage this does and how it makes the chemicals in the plastic bottles unstable.

Never drink bottled water that has been stored in the sun. A glass bottle or stainless steel flask is a better option to carry water. You can also purchase a bottle made from corn which is safe, especially for children, where carrying glass bottles to school is not an option. They are inexpensive, reusable and reclyclable.

143

These corn reusable sources have much less impact on the environmental than plastic water bottles which is an important factor for the next generation. If you drink from a particular bottle, wash it thoroughly to stop bacteria building up.

Much of the information I have given here is underreported in the media, but it is obvious that we need to open our eyes to this information and educate ourselves about the dangers that these potentially harmful chemicals pose to our health.

What is the solution?

It is so easy to clean the water coming into your home – no matter what your budget is. Nothing is more important for you and your family's health than clean water and this short guide will help you evaluate three different types of home filtration systems that are easily available. As a cost comparison, I have picked an economically priced distiller, a reasonably priced reverse-osmosis system and a more up-market atmospheric purification system. After the initial outlay, I am sure you will find no comparison in the cost of bottled water versus that of installing a home-filtration system. All in all, it saves a lot of money in the long term – and you will have the peace of mind knowing you and your family are drinking safe water.

Distilled water

This is one of the most effective – and cheapest – ways to remove chemicals and purify water. Distillers are used in scientific research institutes and laboratories for sterilising equipment which is a good recommendation of the effectiveness and purity of this type of system. They are simple to operate, do not require installation and are basically maintenance free. The initial outlay is not expensive and consumption of electricity is minimal, which means you get pure water at the lowest possible cost.

The body of the distiller looks rather like a large electric kettle that sits conveniently on a counter top in your kitchen. It is easy to use – you fill the distiller to the water line, plug it in and press a button. As the water is boiled, it kills off any bacteria and viruses present. The water is then vaporised to disperse bacteria, chemicals and other contaminants. The vapour is then condensed back into a contaminate-free liquid. This ensures about 99 per cent of your drinking water is pure. Some models shut off automatically when the water boils off, but it is best to time the distiller to finish just before the water boils off to avoid a build-up of mineral deposits in the machine. The machines are easy to clean if you rinse and wipe after use. You will be surprised at the amount of dirt that is left at the bottom of the distiller after processing.

Distillers eliminate the cost and inconvenience of buying bottled mineral water. There have been concerns that distilled water removes minerals from water – and some manufacturers often use this myth to gain an advantage over their competitors. What most people don't realise is that human's best absorb minerals through foods, not water – 95 per cent of the minerals we need come from plants. Plants pick up minerals from the soil and make them available to us.

Reverse osmosis

Reverse osmosis is the home-drinking water system that is most commonly known for its use in converting sea water into drinking water, though they are also made for both mains and well-water sources. It is a filtration method that removes contaminants by passing the water through multiple filters and a semi-permeable membrane. Passing through the various stages produces pure water by screening out the salts and other contaminants. The various filters remove chlorine, fluoride and other chemical contaminants, heavy metals, bacteria, viruses, organic compounds and even radioactive material, which ensures about a 95 per cent purity rate for your drinking water.

A question I am often asked is whether or not water filtered using reverse osmosis is alkaline-forming. Both distilled and reverse osmosis water produce a negative ion reaction in the system, and negative ions are alkaline-forming. Water-treatment plants throughout the world have adopted reverse osmosis as their preferred method of improving water quality.

A reverse osmosis unit sits under your kitchen sink. It connects to a separate tap on your sink and it is also possible to connect to your refrigerator's water supply for making ice. Many people buy one- or two-stage carbon filters systems and expect these to provide clean water, but these cheap systems really only filter out large molecules from the water.

Atmospheric water

This system uses reverse-osmosis technology but requires no water source, which does mean that these systems are limited by atmospheric humidity to some extent. This type of generator extracts water from vapour in the atmosphere and converts it into pure drinking water. Therefore there are none of the problems that are associated with drinking polluted ground water.

They are a good replacement for conventional water coolers in offices as it cuts down on lugging heavy water bottles about and can be used wherever there is an electrical outlet nearby. They are also useful in locations where water is scarce or difficult to obtain, such as dry desert climates. I guess that's something we don't have to worry about in Ireland! The downside is that they come with a sizeable up-front investment as the initial outlay is pretty steep. Also, you will have to factor in the electrical costs as the energy required to drive some of these atmospheric generators can be expensive.

***

Drinking water has many benefits and I encourage you to drink lots of it for the sake of your health, just make sure you know its source.

Key points to remember

- Clean the water coming into your home. This is the first step in drinking clean water.

- If you drink bottled water make sure you know and trust its source. Don't just accept that it is safe.

- Use glass or corn bottles, or a stainless steel flask to carry water. These reusable containers are much better for your health and for the health of our planet.

- Wash reusable bottles thoroughly to stop the build-up of bacteria.

- Get involved with independent groups that are working to improve our water supply. We cannot stick our heads in the sand on these issues, as these groups need your support to lobby government ministers to take action. It may just need an e-mail or a 'like' on Facebook to spread the word to enlighten people as to how they are being misled by public health policy (see www. irelandagainstfluoridation.org).

15

Removing the chemicals from your life

*'I did research when I was pregnant with my first daughter
and was horrified by the chemicals in products, even those
meant for babies.'*

JESSICA ALBA

Have you ever checked the ingredients in the toiletries you use? Many shampoos, toothpastes, deodorants, moisturisers, baby wipes, sunscreens, perfumes and hair dyes contain health-threatening chemicals such as fluoride, sodium lauryl sulphate, propylene glycol, parabens and PABA. Even baby products contain chemicals that you may not wish to use. Inside the tubes and bottles of the beauty products that are part of daily life lurks a cocktail of dangerous synthetic chemicals. Some of the problems associated with using these chemicals are neurotoxicity, developmental toxicity and a weakened immune system.

I have pointed out again and again that advertisers spend a lot of money trying to persuade us that their products are a necessity in our lives. If you are going to part with your cash, you need to find out exactly what you are spending your money on and whether the products are safe for you and your family's health. The manufacturer has a duty to list the ingredients used but it's down to you to check this list and be aware of the harmful ingredients that lurk in many personal-care products.

The list of chemicals that are used in eye make-up, lipstick, shower wash, cleansers, hair sprays, perfumes, baby wipes, sun-screens, fake tan and powders is endless and it is impossible to cover all of them.

Young girls are now reaching puberty at a much younger age than they did 10 to 15 years ago. Research undertaken as part of the University of Bristol's 'Children of the 90s' study suggests that one girl in six reaches puberty before the age of eight. The National Cancer Institute took 1,200 girls aged six to eight to evaluate the age of onset of puberty. They found that 15 per cent of the girls had reached puberty by seven, while more than a quarter of girls had reached puberty by eight years. Doctors are now reporting that girls of six years of age are reaching menstruation. One of the suspected reasons for this dramatic change in the onset of puberty is phthalates – compounds that are found in perfumes, nail polish, air fresheners, detergents and cleaning products. Pthallate compounds can also be found in water and the food chain. They disrupt the delicate balance of hormones as they mimic oestrogen's effects on body tissue.

The question is: How can we avoid the toxic chemicals that are abundant in the pretty packaged jars and bottles that line our bathroom shelves? Well it is relatively easy to reduce your exposure to hazardous chemicals of common beauty products, you simply buy a safer product. There are lots of them out there to choose from (see the Resources section).

Many manufacturers offer a full range of natural hair care, deodorants, toothpastes, shampoos, lipsticks, make-up and skin-care products that are formulated from natural extracts of solvent-free oils, such as aloe vera, chamomile, Shea butter, sesame and jojoba and rosehip oils. Natural products assist in balancing the skin's natural oils, leaving it soft, nourished and hydrated. On sensitive, fragile skin, these natural oils work wonders and many of them give a rich vitamin E antioxidant boost, which is really beneficial to ageing skin.

Harsh chemical products may cause inflammation and eczema when they come into contact with the skin, so choose products that are made from trusted ingredients, those where you are confident of the manufacturer's assurance of the purity and quality. Take note of all the ingredients, so there are no hidden surprises.

Of course, very few of us have time to scrutinise and check labels especially when we are confronted with a list of complicated chemical ingredients. There are literally thousands of chemicals that are used in personal-care products, but let's keep this list as clear and uncomplicated as possible so the next time you purchase some toiletries you will know exactly what to watch out for.

Toothpaste

Toothpaste that contains fluoride and sodium lauryl sulphate, which contains carcinogenic properties that are toxic to human health. Scientists have linked fluoride to dental fluorosis, arthritis, allergic reactions, neurological damage and cancer. Despite this fact, some dentists still recommend toothpastes that contain these ingredients to prevent cavities. Dental fluorosis (permanent pitting and discolouration on the enamel of teeth) is not what you'd expect from a toothpaste.

First let me say that the cause of dental cavities is a lack of good oral hygiene and a diet rich in sugars. I have written enough about the dangers of fluoride in Chapter 14 on water (see page 138), but I remind you again that fluoride is a dangerous poison that can build up in your tissues and cause neurological damage.

Sodium lauryl sulphate (SLS) is another ingredient found in many toothpastes. This is a harsh chemical that is harmful to skin tissue – it is used in laboratories to irritate skin on animals to test healing agents. In toothpastes and shampoos, it is used as a foaming agent.

On top of this, many types of toothpaste contain sodium saccharin which is added for sweetness. This artificial sweetener is a well-known carcinogen (cancer-causing substance).

Triclosan is another highly toxic chemical that is added to toothpaste for its anti-bacterial properties. The Environmental Protection Agency (EPA) in America has recently registered it as a dangerous pesticide that poses a risk to human health and the environment. Tufts University School of Medicine in Boston has also examined triclosan in relation to human health and safety.

Believe it or not, if you buy toothpaste in America, it comes with a warning that states clearly: 'If more than what is needed for brushing is accidentally swallowed, contact a poisons control centre immediately.'

Surely this is not something we should be putting into our mouths when there are safer alternatives. Check it out for yourself.

Just because you have used these familiar products twice a day over long periods of time don't assume they are safe to use. Do you really want to use toothpaste that contains chemicals that may penetrate through the tissue of your mouth, enter your blood stream, and build up in your kidneys, heart, liver and lungs? Finding a non-toxic alternative is a far safer option than ingesting poisonous chemicals.

Hair dyes

The main ingredients to take note of when buying a hair dye are parabens, ammonia, resorcinol, peroxide and p-Phenylenediamine. Some of these chemicals have been banned in France, Sweden and Germany because of the dangers they pose. Hairdressers may be slow to tell you that some of the chemicals used in hair dye products are reported to be carcinogenic (cancer-causing). Indeed, many of them may be totally unaware of the danger posed from using these products, as well as breathing in their toxic fumes. Despite the fact that some studies have found an increased risk of bladder cancer in hairdressers and barbers, many remain poorly educated about the risks to themselves and their clients.

Educating yourself about the increased risks and finding products that are less damaging is your best defence in avoiding adverse reactions to conventional hair colours. The visible signs of hair loss and allergic reactions are not the only dangers involved. Reproductive toxicity, breathing problems and damage to your organs can result from use of toxic hair colours. Dark hair dyes in particular seem to be more dubious than the lighter shades.

Switching from one brand to another can also pose another risk because the ammonia and toxins that remain in your hair from one product can react with the chemicals in the new hair product. So be careful if you are chopping and changing from one colour to another if you want to avoid unnecessary toxic reactions and hair loss.

One of my readers, Ursula, has coloured her hair for years in an effort to cover her grey hair. She wanted a change of colour and tried a different salon. Although they did a patch test to ensure she was not allergic to the chemicals, she soon began to suffer from an itchy irritation to her eyes and a burning sensation on her scalp. Shortly afterwards, her hair began to fall out in chunks in her hands. As you can imagine, this was beyond distressing for Ursula. She contacted the salon immediately only to be told it was not their fault that she was allergic to the product. Ursula was furious.

When she asked if they could contact the company who had supplied the dye, she discovered that these companies are not obligated by law to test their products and that the products are not regulated for safety. After about a year, and many, many trips to her doctor and having got no satisfaction from the defensive hairdresser, Ursula's hair loss and irritated burning scalp began to clear up. Although her hair began to slowly regrow, Ursula was naturally very reluctant to colour her hair. Now in her early fifties, she was also very self-conscious of her grey hair. It took her some time to find the answer to her problem was a vegetable dye which she now finds does the job nicely.

There are a few alternatives to conventional hair dyes. If you colour your hair on a regular basis, why not try a vegetable dye? These colours do not cause the same allergic reactions as the conventional dyes that are full of synthetic chemicals. Plus they are not as harsh on your hair. Some salons use herbal formulations that are odour and chemical free.

Beware of salons that have poor ventilation, as there may be high levels of toxic fumes in the air that you may well be breathing in. Reducing this exposure to toxic chemical fumes is not just good for the customer but also the staff who may have worked with highly toxic chemicals for a number of years. Check out salons in your area to see if you can find one that is aware of these issues. Don't be shy. Do your homework. It's up to you to ask questions and find a safe method to colour your hair. Protecting your health makes sense.

Deodorants

Given the widespread, repeated use of deodorants, this is another product that must be looked at closely. You would do well to avoid deodorants that contain aluminium salts and parabens. Most of us assume these pretty packaged toiletries are safe to use, but unfortunately this is not always the case. Deodorants kill off the bacteria that cause unpleasant odours to develop. When you spray antiperspirant deodorants directly onto your armpits, it blocks your sweat ducts and stops you from sweating.

Your body is designed to sweat. Perspiration is one of the natural routes of detoxification from the lymphatic system. If you block the detoxification process, toxins may build up in your lymph glands.

Aluminium salts is the main ingredient that is used to block sweat ducts. These salts are then absorbed through the skin. Aluminium is a neurotoxin that builds up in the brain, liver and lungs and directly affects these delicate organs. It has been linked to the growth of cancerous cells in the breast because it can mimic the activity of the hormone oestrogen. It is thought that it disrupts the production of natural oestrogen by the body. Many deodorants also contain harsh chemicals such as sodium lauryl sulphates and triethanolamine.

Another point to remember is when you shave it is much easier for chemicals to enter your body, as shaving strips away some of the protective outer layer of the skin.

Over the years, I have used many different deodorants before finally settling on one that is aluminium and parabens free. It's a lovely blend of tangerine, mandarin and lavender oils, combined with vanilla extract that contains no harsh ingredients. It leaves me smelling and feeling fresh and clean throughout the day and gives me the all-day protection I need.

Shampoo

Sodium lauryl sulphates (SLS) and sodium laureth sulfate (SLES) are found in most shampoos – some have concentrations of up to 30 per cent – but they have long-lasting effects on the liver.

As SLS is a corrosive skin irritant, it can cause cataracts in adults. It is found in baby shampoos, even the 'no more tears' varieties. 'No more tears' may sound quite appealing at first, but you may not relish the thought quite so much when you consider that this substance can prevent children's eyes from developing properly.

The Campaign for Safe Cosmetics found some baby shampoos in America tested positive for the compounds 1,4-dioxane and formaldehyde which are suspected carcinogens and common skin and eye irritants. These chemicals are not listed on the bottle as an added ingredient but when the other chemicals are mixed 1,4-dioxane is created. This makes it difficult for the consumer to decipher whether the product is safe to use.

Manufacturers often claim that the quantities are too small to raise alarm. Isn't it just easier to source a shampoo that does not contain these harmful substances?

Skin care, baby wipes and sunscreens

The skin is a key organ of the body, with a unique trans-dermal delivery system that transports molecules into the bloodstream. The speed with which this can happen was demonstrated by a Danish study of healthy male volunteers who applied cosmetic creams containing parabens. The skin's unique ability to absorb and diffused the molecules of the cream across membranes led to the detection of dangerous substances in their bloodstreams within an hour.

Propylene glycol and parabens are the offending substances found in skin care products. The EDF (Environmental Defense

Fund) in America has listed these compounds as a suspected neurotoxicity hazard as they also have the ability to cause kidney damage and liver abnormalities.

***

When you consider that, on average, we use at least eight different personal-care products each day – from toothpaste, shampoo, conditioner, body wash or soap, deodorant, cologne and moisturisers – you realise the potential for these chemicals to enter our bloodstreams. In many cases, women use a heck of a lot more of these potentially harmful chemical products than men. If there were tighter regulations on the chemical industry, the worst of these chemicals would be phased out and replaced.

It makes real sense to reduce your exposure to the invisible dangers of harsh chemical products. It is incredibly easy to adopt a new skincare regime – simply buy a safer alternative that won't weaken your immune system.

Key points to remember

- Less is best. Fewer chemicals mean less exposure.

- Avoid toothpaste that contains fluoride and sodium lauryl sulphate as they carry carcinogenic properties that are toxic to human health. Also watch out for sodium saccharin and triclosan. If your toothpaste contains any of these ingredients, change it.

- Avoid deodorants that contain aluminium salts and parabens. Don't apply deodorant after shaving as shaving strips away some of the protective outer layer of the skin.

- If you want to revitalise your hair, check all shampoos for sodium lauryl sulphate and sodium laureth sulfate.

- Ask your hairdresser if the hair dyes they use contain parabens, ammonia, resorcinol, peroxide or p-Phenylenediamine. If the answer is yes, change the hair dye or the hairdresser.

- Skin care, baby wipes and sunscreens should all be free of propylene glycol and parabens. Your skin deserves the best.

- Don't assume you can trust the manufacturer's claims of 'natural', 'pure' and 'hyper-allergenic'. Do you research and find a range of products that will work for you and your family.

- Keep this short list at hand when you go shopping it will help you eliminate some of the chemicals from your life.

- Throw away all the toiletries that have harmful ingredients.

- If you don't make the switch, you should at least bear in mind the real cost of a weakened immune system when applying chemical products to your body.

16

Signing up for fun

'People rarely succeed unless they have fun in what they are doing.'

DALE CARNEGIE

I am a firm believer that physical activities must be fun if we are to encourage people to leave the telly and comfy sofa to exercise their butts off. There is little to say about exercise other than it is a vital part of our physical wellbeing, so it would be remiss of me not to address the subject. Let's face it, most of us shy away from strenuous exercise but, when it comes down to it, there are no two ways about it *your body needs it*. Although this may be blindingly obvious, most of us view exercise only as a weight-control measure, but exercise keeps all the mechanical parts of the body in good working order.

Let's look briefly at some of the benefits physical exercise has on the body. Most importantly, it brings oxygen into the bloodstream, increasing the flow of energy around the body. This is especially useful for the passive lymph system which unlike the blood system (heart) does not have a pump. As the lymph system is a major system for detoxification within the body, it's essential to move it regularly. Exercise also eliminates the build-up of cholesterol in arteries, diminishes the risk of diabetes, stroke and heart disease, and mops up free radicals. Now that can't be bad.

It's also worth pointing out that we also benefit emotionally from exercise, as it releases endorphins (happy hormones) that reduce stress, anxiety and lift depression. I think we could all do with a bit of that, don't you? Exercise will put the 'oomph' back in your life. Don't forget that regular exercise gives you stamina and flexibility, not to mention confidence – all important in many areas of your life, including your love life.

While trying to persuade you of the importance of a fitness regime, you might have many excuses – I'm too tired, it's boring, I simply don't have the time – it's one of the things you'll get around to or perhaps you are the I'll-start-tomorrow type. It's a very human tendency.

Now, I understand that in today's fast-paced world we are all subject to time constraints and so the discipline of a fitness regime may not be high on your agenda. If this is the case, you can probably think of a thousand things you could be doing and exercise is not one of them. But if you're looking in the mirror in horror, or you find that you're always tired, your body may be crying out for a bit of attention, it may well be time for you to step up and raise your game. In the words of Willis Whitney:

Some men have thousands of reasons why they cannot do what they want to, when all they need is one reason why they can.

The vast majority of us resolve that we will exercise more, especially if we have an event coming up. We make solid promises that we will get our act together and won't collapse in a heap on the couch every evening. This is because we are focused on the outcome as opposed to the pain. We picture how we will look in that outfit or on the beach, etc. Instead of getting fit and healthy just for an occasion, wouldn't it be great if you had a longer term sustainable goal that you could keep in mind? It could be something like being fit enough to play tennis with your children or having the kind of body that clothes look well on all the time.

I know many of us yearn for the days when fitness never seemed to be an issue, when we did not have to spend time trying to keep slim, trim and fit. The crux of the problem, when it comes to exercising, is the way we view working out. The mere thoughts of 'no pain, no gain' and 'feeling the burn' puts us right off. It leaves us feeling tired out long before we hit the gym. This is a misguided idea because pain is usually a signal that you are doing something wrong. Start with gentle exercise and build slowly. While any amount of exercise is worthwhile, you need a minimum of twenty minutes at a good pace, where you are slightly out of breath (and ideally a bit sweaty) before you start to burn fat. So if weight is an issue, that's your absolute minimum.

A couple of encouraging facts for you: you continue to burn calories for between twelve and twenty-four hours after exercising. The more muscle you have, the more calories you burn even when you are idle.

The mind plays a major role in your success with exercise. If you dread getting started, there is no doubt you are going to find it tough. This is not an attitude problem, more the perception problem. Exercise will always represent a challenge if it is hindered by a perception of hard work and pain. The source of the confusion is our failure to distinguish between attitude and perception. Of course, that could be because of the many vain attempts we've made at exercising in the past.

This could be the real reason why we are slow to give exercising another shot, as we all judge ourselves on past experiences. First of all, change your old way of thinking – it will help tremendously and shift your energy to a much more positive state. If you have a negative view of exercise, you are likely to pack it in at the first sign of a stiff limb or sore muscle. When you were a kid, you did not exercise you played, so *play* golf, tennis, soccer or basketball or whatever game you enjoy. There are so many forms of exercise out there that there is bound to be one that appeals to you. I can only really tell you about those that I have tried.

Exercising can change things for the better. It can help you get more out of life. If you are still wondering what's the point, why not just kick off with a bit of fun? The worst-case scenario is that you might end up with a stiff limb or a sore muscle. I know everybody's idea of a workout routine is different, but you don't have to be an adventure junkie to drag your butt off the couch.

Don't imagine I am some sort of shining example of human fitness. There are days I struggle to get motivated to exercise as much as the next person. All I ask is that you do something – don't just sit there. The plan is to get you fit and healthy and this requires you to muck in a bit. It will be worth it in the end. So are you up for a bit of a challenge? Come on, there is a multitude of things you can try.

Walking or hiking

To start the ball rolling, you could try getting out for a simple walk. It's a great way of eliminating toxins from the body. The important thing to do is to keep a good pace so that you are slightly breathless. Think of the money you'll save on those expensive gym fees although you may need a serious pair of runners if you are to be comfortable. Walking in the fresh air is a great way to get started and good for people who don't like gyms.

Research has shown that most people feel a boost in their well-being after a walk. It is a great motivator to have a friend to tag along with you, and you are far more likely to go the distance and not give in if you have a pal with you. Make sure they have similar goals so that you both stay focused on the exercise. For me, I tend to slow down to make sure I have enough breath to chat when I am with some of my buddies. There is a possible flipside to depending on someone else to motivate you – if they have to cancel, you may cry off too. Choose your exercise buddy wisely or go it alone, but do get out there. Oh yeah, and the weather is never a good excuse to cancel. If you are waiting for the ideal weather, you may never do much outdoors. Get yourself a decent jacket and go for it. Give it a go for a week and I guarantee that by the Friday you will feel the benefit.

Have some fun in the gym

How about joining a gym? You may believe you're time enough getting into all that when you really have to or maybe you're not the *gym* type.

In a gym, you can choose between classes, swimming or circuit training, so you can vary it to keep it interesting. Join competitions or charity fitness fundraisers, train with friends – whatever it takes to motivate you. If you are working with a fitness trainer, make sure they know what your goals are and update the trainer as your goals change. As you achieve your goals, you will need new ones so that you are constantly motivated. Include the machines or exercises that are fun for you as well as those that are simply essential to achieve a healthy body.

You are destined to fail if you don't enjoy it and then you may spend your time feeling guilty about the empty promises you made to yourself. That certainly won't produce the body you've always dreamed of, whereas a toned, fit body could well be in sight if you are prepared to step up and give it a go. Exercise should be fun. It's not a punishment for weight that you have gained. Joining a gym could be just the helping hand you need, you will mix with others who have the same interests and you will have a trainer to give your specific needs some time and attention.

If you can't afford to join a gym, get yourself an exercise video and either a few weights or resistance bands or maybe a skipping rope. That's more than enough to get you started. Don't forget to do different exercises each day to work different muscles in your body and to give those you worked excessively the previous day a break.

Massage

This may not sound much like exercise to you, but I am hoping to entice you into releasing those happy hormones. A good massage is a very nice treat that will get you relaxed and invigorated. Massage is wonderful for the lymphatic system which is one of the body's defence mechanisms. The lymph system filters out organisms that cause disease, produces certain white blood cells and generates antibodies. It is also important for the distribution of fluids and nutrients in the body, because it drains excess fluids and protein so tissues do not swell up.

Many therapists shy away from massaging people with health challenges, especially people with cancer. That is more to do with their fear that massage is contraindicated for people with cancer because it may help spread the disease. Although this notion is still pervasive amongst many therapists, it is possible to find some who have a good knowledge base and specialise in this important immune booster. Try a massage, it is a wonderful way to improve circulation, restore energy and reduce pain. It's heavenly and it will rejuvenate your spirits and make you feel relaxed.

Watch television

Have I got your attention? Exercise is not a punishment so if you're finding it hard to get yourself off the sofa try stretching in front of the telly. You can also try some sit-ups or lifting small weights while watching a movie or your favourite soap. It may seem like a lazy way to go about it, but it will get your body moving. If you have limited mobility, this is a gentle way to get started. Perhaps you can then move on to the Wii exercise games or their equivalent.

Weight lifting

Of all the gadgets we supposedly need to keep fit, a set of weights is probably the best investment of all. Lifting weights is essential if you are to maintain healthy bones. A small set of weights won't set you back much and won't take up too much space. However, make sure you buy a set that's heavy enough for your needs as you want to challenge your muscles to lift more weight. Build up the repetitions gradually and you will soon see results – you don't have to become an Olympic champion. Lifting weights two to three times a week will maintain healthy bone structure and stave off osteoporosis.

Aerobics

If aerobic exercise leaves you wheezing and out of breath, the best advice I can give you is to invest in a good DVD this will encourage you to *just do it* at home. It's a must if you want to stay motivated. It's like your own personal trainer. A good DVD will push you a bit harder that you would yourself, so you accomplish more in a shorter time. My son tells me he is far more inclined to work out when he has a few tunes to listen to, he says it takes the chore out of it, but you don't have to brave the lashing rain and the music will also help you take it one step farther. You also have the added bonus of being able to decide when you have the time and you don't need to stick to schedules.

Running

Well, I'm afraid, running solo is not my idea of fun, though I have great admiration for those committed joggers I see pounding the pavements in all kinds of weather in my local village. One of my friends jogs with her seven-month-old baby, she has one of those designer buggies and, I must say, she looks incredibly trendy, kitted out in all the gear. She finds it a great way to stop her baby whining and she gets the benefits of keeping fit.

Runners keep telling me about the natural high that they get due to the endorphins they release after a good run. Maybe I should try it.

Cycling

I must say I love cycling. It's great fun heading off to the park and getting a bit of fresh air into the bargain. Even if you, or your bike, are a bit rusty, I am sure you will enjoy shifting into gear and turning exercise into some carefree fun.

Swimming

Swimming is a super, non-impact exercise, but I must admit since I began swimming in salt-water pools and ozone treated pool on holidays, I can't bring myself to take the plunge in chlorinated pools anymore. Chlorine is defined as a gaseous, poisonous, corrosive chemical that combines with nearly every other element. It is widely used as a disinfectant, so my natural inclination is to steer clear of it. Besides, it can wreak havoc with your hair. This one is not for me. Mind you, there's always the sea!

Dancing

Spontaneity can be fun, doing things on the spur of the moment is exciting. So why not just do something totally unplanned? How about dancing? I can't think of a better way to knock off a few pounds. Dancing not only enables you to exercise, you get to have great fun at the same time. I joined Zumba classes with my daughter Julie and it would do your heart good to see the girls in their late sixties mixed in with all the teenagers. Even if you believe you have two left feet or are not ultra-co-ordinated, you can bend all the rules you want while dancing. It will keep you looking your best and will help you stay young at heart. Turning exercise into fun produces an abundance of endorphins. I say, bring it on.

Yoga

The ancient practice of yoga helps promote good health and inner peace. At first when I began to practise yoga, I found it very slow – but one of the reasons for this is that I chose the wrong type of yoga! There are several types to choose from. Hot yoga is the fastest growing form of yoga in the world and is suitable for all levels of ability. Hatha yoga is a Westernised form of yoga that is slow-paced stretching with some simple breathing exercises and seated meditation. Ashtanga yoga is a very fast-moving form of yoga, whereas Iyengar yoga places a lot of emphasis on alignment.

Make sure you choose the one that is right for you. Yoga offers many benefits, like increased flexibility, suppleness and improved muscle tone. Whether you're a novice or experienced the benefits of all that stretching and relaxation are not to be missed. Yoga is suitable for all ages. I recently met a wonderful lady who was 81 years old and who had practised yoga for years. Its benefits are many so go ahead give it a try.

Pilates

If you have not yet managed to find the ideal exercise, why not try Pilates? At least it does not require you to break into a sweat let alone turned purple in the face. It seems to me like a cross between yoga and physiotherapy. No matter what your weight, age or fitness level, this one is simple.

Tai chi

Tai chi consists of precise movements designed to raise energy levels. It's quite a meditative form of exercise. Health, strength and vigour are just some of the benefits of this ancient practice.

Rebounding

I saved the best till last. If you want to sign up for some serious fun, this one gets my vote. Rebounding is a fantastic form of exercise. It improves the lymph system and blood circulation, lowers blood pressure, and raises energy levels. My best investment was a small, fold-away trampoline. You don't need to become a gymnast because you just bounce. Irrespective of age, you will feel you have turned back the clock when you're rebounding. You cannot patent the fun you will have. If nothing else, it will make you smile. It's the perfect exercise and I guarantee it's fun and my word will you feel alive. Sound too good to be true? Well don't take my word for it, give it a go.

***

Don't file these activities under your to do list – remember that actions speak louder than words. Enjoy the results.

Key points to remember

- Find something you enjoy that will encourage you to be active. It will stack the odds in your favour.

- Look forward to your work out with enthusiasm. Don't think of it in a negative way.

- Get yourself a workout partner. A pal will take your mind off exercise and help you maintain a regular practice. Thank heavens for friends.

- Focus on those great abs, that tight bum and the increased energy you will enjoy. That will spur you on to success.

- Turn on some tunes to keep you motivated. Music will help you perform better over a longer period of time.

- Join a gym – if you can't afford the gym fees, invest in an exercise DVD. Then you will have your very own personal instructor.

- Stay hydrated while working out. A drop in body fluids leads to a loss in energy levels. Drink plenty of water but stay away from energy drinks that will spike your blood sugars and rob your energy.

- Whatever you do, stay active. What could be more important than a healthy, toned, fit body?

- Go on, release those happy hormones!

17

Transition and therapeutic recipes

'Let food be thy medicine, thy medicine shall be thy food.'

HIPPOCRATES

For simplicity in this section, I have separated the recipes into two groups: transition recipes and therapeutic recipes.

Transition recipes

Those recipes marked 'transition' are for those of you who want to make changes to improve your health but who are not facing a health challenge. These recipes include fruits and potatoes which are omitted from the therapeutic recipes.

If you are just starting to juice, you can mix fruits with veggies. The sweet fruits will encourage a good juicing regime and, as you progress, you can gradually phase out the fruits in favour of vegetables. Be aware that fructose from fruits will spike your blood-sugar levels even though they are natural sugars. Add some water to dilute the sugar content of the juice. All you will need is just some fresh fruits and vegetables, a good juicer and the commitment of time to make two juices each day.

Potatoes are nightshades that contain a substance called alkaloids. Alkaloids can impact on joints and nerve-muscle function. So if you have arthritic problems, they are not the best food for you.

These recipes will help you successfully transition to a healthier diet without having to starve yourself or feel deprived. All of the therapeutic recipes can also be used by those going through the transition phase.

Therapeutic recipes

The 'therapeutic' recipes are for those of you who want to lose weight or who are facing a health challenge. They are a bit more hard core. I have chosen these particular recipes because they won't spike your blood sugars and so they don't increase weight gain or encourage the growth of fungus, yeasts, parasites or cancer.

Eating nutritious foods is a very effective way to create a body that is resistant to disease. Mother Nature has laced thousands of foods with nutrients that help keep infections and other illnesses at bay. Eating these nutritious foods will ultimately mean better health and fewer trips to your doctor. The therapeutic recipes will also help you lose unwanted weight permanently without depriving yourself. There are some recipes from some of my favourite chefs in Dublin from Cornucopia and Nautulis for the more adventurous.

Remember that this a lifestyle change and not just a sexy temporary diet that has no lasting results. Even the smallest change can help you break harmful habits and create better ones. Small and attainable steps can have a big impact on your life. Many people only change their eating habits when they are forced to because of a health issue. Don't wait or put it off for the right time – the right time is now. The *Eat Yourself Well* formula is to keep it simple and start today.

Juices and smoothies

Juices are a wonderful way to recharge your batteries and boost your immune system. It is my absolute number-one recommendation to improve your health. Juices have antioxidant and anti-inflammatory components, as well as essential enzymes, vitamins and minerals which help keep all kinds of ailments and diseases at bay. Health challenges don't just magically disappear, you have to make an effort, and there's no better way to do this than with some delicious juices.

As juices hydrate the body, you can easily cut out empty calories from soft drinks that contain artificial sweeteners. Chemical sweeteners in diet soft drinks acidify the body and cause you to retain fluids, giving you a bloated appearance. Carbonated soft drinks contain phosphoric acid which accelerates bone loss. Remember nothing can replace the wonderful foods that Mother Nature has given to us. Besides, think of the money you'll save on soft drinks and carton juices which lose their beneficial enzymes in the pasteurisation process.

If you are looking for a quick pick-me-up to overcome fatigue and a lack of energy, juicing will give you that new lease of life you have been looking for. I hope these mouth-watering recipes will inspire you to get juicing. Remember, all of the therapeutic recipes can also be used by those who are in the transition phase.

Bottoms up!

1. **Turbo-charge your immune system (therapeutic)**
2. **Anti-ageing juice (therapeutic)**
3. **Sparkling mojitos (therapeutic)**
4. **Zingy lemonade (therapeutic)**
5. **Irresistible mocktails (transition)**
6. **Afternoon energiser (transition)**
7. **Good-fat shake (transition)**
8. **Sugar blues smoothie (transition)**
9. **Frothy and fresh (transition)**

∽ *Turbo-charge your immune system (therapeutic)* ∽

Wheatgrass is one of the most nutrient-dense, vitamin-packed plants nature has to offer. It has a very distinctive taste which not all palates appreciate. Ginger will not totally mask the unfamiliar taste fully, but it does complement it ever so delicately in the background. Wheatgrass boosts your energy reserves to overflowing, especially if you are feeling rundown, sluggish or lethargic. Some people report that it gives them a buzz similar to caffeine, without the unwanted side-effects. You can grow your own or buy online (see the Resources section).

Serves 1

> *'If you want to turbo charge your immune system and energy levels, I encourage you to try this one.'*

I shot of wheatgrass

¼ inch piece of ginger or a squeeze of lemon

Crushed ice (optional)

Directions

1. Cut and wash a third of a tray of wheatgrass. Put the ginger and grass through the juicer and process.

2. Pour over some crushed ice if you like.

ᔋ *Anti-ageing juice (therapeutic)* ᔋ

This anti-ageing juice staves off free-radical damage in the body and slows down the ageing process. Kale is packed with chlorophyll, and consuming foods that are rich in chlorophyll is important if you want to look and feel younger. Ginger is great aid for digestive problems. Cucumbers hydrate and clean the body. This green juice helps to clean out the intestines and remove harmful waste from the colon.

Serves 1–2

'This is a powerful cleansing and healing juice. I use it on a regular basis.'

1 cucumber

2 celery stalks

A handful of kale or parsley

1 small chunk of ginger

Directions

1. Process all ingredients through the juicer. If the cucumber is large enough, this recipe will serve two people.

❦ *Sparkling mojitos (therapeutic)* ❦

If you are in a party mood or feel like rewarding yourself, this non-alcoholic mojito is a winner. I find this too sweet for my taste, but I know many people who have acquired a taste for mojitos and cannot seem to get enough them. For those of you who fall into this category, this alcohol-free drink is very easy to whisk up. Our guests love them.

Serves 2

*'On the bright side, you won't have a hangover
in the morning.'*

1 cup of lime juice

2 cups of sparkling water

1 handful of mint leaves

10 drops of stevia

2 handfuls of crushed ice

Directions

1. Blend the lime juice, stevia and mint leaves together.

2. Pour over the crushed ice in two cocktail glasses and add the sparkling water.

3. Stir everything together.

⤜ *Zingy lemonade (therapeutic)* ⤛

If you want to waken up your taste buds, this refreshing lemonade is for you. Home-made lemonade is usually made by dissolving sugar in hot water to disperse the sugar granules through the lemonade, but this recipe is sugar free. Heat it slightly in the winter months or add some ice to create a refreshing thirst-quencher in the summer.

Serves 2

'Lemons cleanse and detoxify the body. They are also very effective at cleaning the palate.'

I cup of lemon juice

4 cups of cold water

15 drops of stevia

2 cups of ice cubes

Lemon slices (to serve)

Directions

1. Add the juice, liquid stevia and water to a jug to the desired strength. If the lemonade is not sweet enough for your taste, add a little more stevia to the mix.

⤚ *Irresistible mocktails (transition)* ⤚

Whether you are looking for a refreshing drink or you fancy a mocktail, here's an easy one for you. Although this drink has no alcohol, be assured it is not lacking in taste. If you love cocktails but don't want the alcohol (or are abstaining for health reasons) try this fabulous drink. It's a nice alternative for a treat or for party guests who prefer not to drink alcohol if they are driving.

Serves 1–2

'You won't feel left out, you will feel right in with the cocktail scene.'

I grapefruit

I cup of cranberries

I cup of sparkling water

10 drops of stevia

Dash of lime

Handful of crushed ice

Directions

1. Juice the grapefruit and cranberries.

2. Add the stevia, sparking water and lime.

3. Pour over crushed ice.

∽ *Afternoon energiser (transition)* ∽

If you are short on energy and want to recharge your batteries mid-afternoon, this juice will do the trick. The ingredients are easy to find, but do try your best to buy organic. If you cannot source organic fruit and veggies then peel the ones you have. Carrots are rich in beta-carotene, which is great for the eyes as carotenoids help keep UV rays from damaging the eyes and causing cataracts. They are also rich in absorbable calcium, whereas the calcium in many synthetic supplements is secreted by the body because it cannot be absorbed.

Serves 1

'Not only is this juice good for bone health, it will give you a boost of energy so you can avoid the dreaded afternoon slump.'

2 carrots

I apple (including seeds)

¼ lime with skin

Directions

1. Simply wash the ingredients, juice them and you're ready to go.

∽ *Good-fat shake (transition)* ∽

Chia seeds are a healthy addition to shakes and are a great way to add good fats to your diet, they are rich in antioxidants and a good source of omega-3. Soak the chia seeds overnight and add to smoothies or porridge. Alternatively, the ground seeds can be sprinkled on cereals. Udo's oil can also be used in smoothies – it is a rich source of good fats and is wonderful for your skin and hair. So easy!

Serves 1

'Lack of essential fats can lead to cravings as the body needs a regular supply of good fats from foods in order to thrive.'

1 banana

½ cup of almond milk

Small handful of spinach leaves

1 teaspoon of Udo's oil or ½ teaspoon of Chia seeds (soaked)

Ice (to serve)

Directions

1. Blend all ingredients together until smooth.

2. Pour over some ice.

⟨ *Sugar blues smoothie (transition)* ⟩

If you have the sugar blues and simply cannot pacify your sweet tooth, this smoothie is sure to chase them away. Having a sweet alternative in the transition phase will help wean you off sugar. Learning to manage blood-sugar irregularities will mean you won't give in to cravings. Strawberries and raspberries are at their best when they are in season. If you want to improve your skin, strawberries are amazing. They help promote the production of collagen which is a part of the connective tissue that helps the elasticity and constant renewal of skin cells. Raspberries clear out nasal passages of mucus.

Serves 1–2

'The secret with this self-indulgent drink is not to have too many refills.'

¼ cup of strawberries

¼ cup of raspberries

¼ cup of pure water

3 drops of stevia

Handful of ice

Directions

1. Bend all the ingredients until the desired consistency is reached.
2. Add ice and serve.

⤳ *Frothy and fresh (transition)* ⤳

It can be difficult to change our views about dairy because we have been taught throughout our whole lives that milk is a healthy food. But this frothy smoothie, filled with pineapple and coconut milk, will help convince you. The thick creamy coconut milk gives a rich flavour and a creamy texture to this delicious smoothie.

Serves 1–2

'Add a touch of decadence by placing a decorative slice of pineapple on the top of the glass.'

½ pineapple (peeled)

½ cup of tinned coconut milk (400ml)

½ teaspoon of Udo's oil

Handful of ice

Directions

1. Blend all the ingredients until the desired consistency is reached.

2. Add a handful of ice and stir.

Breakfasts and milks

With the dangers associated with cow's milk, it's well worth having a shot at making your own milk. These delicious milks are great alternatives for those who are lactose intolerant or who are simply trying to stay away from dairy products.

You can always juice or have a smoothie for breakfast, but if you prefer a cereal-based breakfast try some of these. Don't be afraid to try new foods, like raw bee pollen, or grains, like buckwheat. You can change the recipes so that you don't get bored and add your own favourite flavours to mix it up a bit. These foods are a nourishing, wholesome and satisfying way to start out your day.

1. **Energy milk (therapeutic)**

2. **Creamy coconut milk (therapeutic)**

3. **Relax and revive (therapeutic)**

4. **Easy peesy yoghurt (therapeutic)**

5. **Raw power breakfast (therapeutic)**

6. **Oatmeal with blueberries (transition)**

7. **Nutty muesli (transition)**

⟿ *Energy milk (therapeutic)* ⟿

Energy is the by-product of eating food, and nut or grain milks are a great food. When you consider the risks associated with dairy milk, it's worth making the switch to alternative sources of milk. I like to use almonds as they have a nice flavour and creamy texture. Add some stevia to give it a hint of sweetness.

'Nut milks are packed with protein and can be used for smoothies or cereals.'

1 cup of pre-soaked almonds

2–3 cups of pure water

3 drops of stevia (optional)

Directions

1. Soak the nuts overnight in water. Rinse and strain off the soak water and discard.

2. Blend all the ingredients in a blender until mixed.

3. Strain through a fine mesh sieve or nut-milk bag or muslin.

4. Retain the pulp as it can be added to cookies or pâté. The milk will last for two or three days when refrigerated.

ꙥ *Creamy coconut milk (therapeutic)* ꙥ

I know it may seem like work to make your own milk, but coconut has many health benefits because of its fibre and nutritional content. The colour and rich taste of the milk can be attributed to the high oil content – and it's the oil that makes coconut a truly remarkable food and medicine. This milk has a faint smell of coconut and the stevia adds a touch of sweetness. It can be used in tea and coffee, poured over cereals or added to soups. You can even bake with it if you are vegan or lactose intolerant.

To make 1 litre

> *'The milk gives a lovely authentic flavour to curries and Indian dishes. Go on you deserve the best.'*

1 200-gram pack of creamed coconut

1 litre of pure water

10 drops of stevia

Directions

1. Put the coconut cream into a blender with half of the water. The water should be added gradually until it blends with the coconut.

2. Add the rest of the water until it becomes a smooth creamy milk.

∽ *Relax and revive (therapeutic)* ∽

Winter brings a change in weather that we can all become more susceptible to colds, influenza and respiratory illness. Bolster yourself against the chill with this delicious oat milk. I add some vanilla extract and cinnamon, which makes a really nice combination and is a good alternative to sugar. Cinnamon has many medicinal uses and helps with colds, nausea, diarrhoea and painful menstrual cramps. Relax and put your feet up.

Serves 1

> *'The rolled cinnamon sticks can be grated into warm drinks or the ground powder sprinkled over the oat milk to relax and revive you in the winter months.'*

I cup of rolled oats

2–3 cups of pure water

3 drops of vanilla extract

Ground or grated cinnamon

Directions

1. Blend all the ingredients in a blender until mixed.

2. Strain through a fine mesh sieve or nut-milk bag. The milk will last for two or three days when refrigerated.

3. Sprinkle with cinnamon.

❧ *Easy peesy yoghurt (therapeutic)* ❧

I like to make my own non-dairy yoghurt. You can also add a good probiotic to the mix to ensure you get a daily dose of good bacteria. Many of the probiotic yoghurts you can buy in the supermarket are loaded with sugars, which encourages the growth of harmful bacteria. The creamed coconut is easily sourced in supermarkets and health stores.

Serves 2

'When you make your own yoghurt, you won't have to worry about added sugars or your waistline.'

½ cup of pure water

1 200-gram pack of creamed coconut

½ teaspoon of vanilla extract

10 drops of stevia

Directions

1. Place all the ingredients into a blender and blend until you get the consistency of creamy yogurt.

2. Add a little extra water until you get the desired consistency.

3. Pour over your favourite breakfast or enjoy on its own.

∽ *Raw power breakfast (therapeutic)* ∽

Buckwheat is related to rhubarb, not wheat, and so is gluten-free. Buckwheat is loaded with an impressive array of useful minerals, such as calcium, iron, magnesium, potassium, zinc, copper, manganese, proteins and antioxidants. It is a powerful grain that is a staple food among the Russian people. This nourishing, wholesome and satisfying breakfast will start out your day on the right footing. You can make several batches at a time and store in a glass container.

Serves 2–4

> *'I add some raw bee pollen to give that delicious sweet hit you need first thing in the morning.'*

2 cups of buckwheat

1 tablespoon of bee pollen

1 cup of oat milk

Directions

1. Soak the buckwheat in water for an hour and then rinse off the starchy soak water.

2. Drain and place the buckwheat on parchment paper on a dehydrator tray.

3. Dry till crunchy and serve with rice or oat milk.

4. Sprinkle bee pollen over the crunchy buckwheat if desired.

➥ *Oatmeal with blueberries (transition)* ➥

As chillier temperatures set in, many people like a warm breakfast to set them on their way. Oats are a good source of soluble and insoluble fibre which sweeps the gut of unwanted waste. Oats are also powerful at reducing blood cholesterol and aiding digestion. Soaking the oats and nuts overnight makes them more digestible and you will soon get into the habit.

Serves 2

> *'You can omit the berries if you are eating from the therapeutic menus and sprinkle with bee pollen.'*

1 cup of flaked oats

1 cup of oat milk

¼ cup of blueberries

¼ cup of chopped hazelnuts

10 drops of stevia (optional)

Directions

1. Soak the flaked oats overnight in oat milk. Also soak the nuts overnight in water (drain and discard the soak water).

2. Warm the oats slightly (in the milk) in a small pot.

3. Serve with the chopped nuts and blueberries.

4. Drizzle some stevia over the top if desired.

⤜ *Nutty muesli (transition)* ⤛

Nourishing, nurturing and protecting ourselves and our immune systems are imperative if we want to achieve optimum health. Sprouted seeds and germinated nuts are loaded with enzymes. When you eat sprouted seeds and nuts, you absorb their nutrients more easily. This breakfast will give you sustainable energy to get you through the morning. Unlike many store-bought mueslis on the market, there are no hidden sugars in this one. You can omit the berries if you are eating from the therapeutic menus.

Serves 1–2

> *'Experiment with different nuts, like pecans or hazelnuts to keep it interesting.'*

1/4 cup of pumpkin seeds

1/4 cup of sunflower seeds

1/3 cup of chopped Brazil nuts

1/2 cup of mixed berries

10 drops of stevia

Directions

1. Soak the seeds and nuts in water overnight. Rinse and drain the following morning, and discard the soak water.

2. Chop the nuts roughly and drizzle with rice, oat or almond milk.

3. Top with the berries and add the stevia.

Soups and starters

If you are looking for culinary inspiration, why not reawaken your taste buds with some different flavours and tastes. There is great joy in exploring new tastes and taking the boredom out of preparing food. I use coconut milks, squash, seaweeds, spices and herbs to add flavour to these easy recipes. I know only too well that there is no joy in spending hours in your kitchen preparing food that neither you nor your family will eat. If you are trying to get the family on board, you need to make food tasty and interesting. The following are tried and tested with my friends and family. I hope you enjoy them.

1. **Rich creamy squash soup (therapeutic)**

2. **Split-pea soup (therapeutic)**

3. **Chilled carrot and avocado soup (therapeutic)**

4. **Fabulous seaweed soup (therapeutic)**

5. **Mushroom pâté with roasted red pepper salsa (therapeutic)**

6. **Omega rich soup (therapeutic)**

7. **Beetroot carpaccio with mustard slaw (transition)**

8. **Mammy's home-made bread (transition)**

9. **Delicious garlic mushrooms (therapeutic)**

ᕙ *Rich creamy squash soup (therapeutic)* ᕙ

I absolutely adore this soup, it is so rich and creamy that you would almost think it was made with full-fat cream. It is great for a dinner party as it can be prepared in advance. I use water to sauté the onion so there is no heating of oils. When oils are heated to high temperatures, they form harmful by-products. For those of you who have never tried squash, this might be the time to give it a go. It will be an instant hit!

Serves 4

'Sprinkle with chopped parsley or basil when serving to add extra colour to this rich and creamy soup.'

1 butternut squash

1 400-ml tin of coconut milk

2 onions

1 tablespoon of vegetable bouillon

1 cup of boiling water

Chopped basil or parsley (for garnish)

Directions

1. Remove the skin and seeds from the squash and peel the onions.

2. Cut the onions and butter squash into slices. Sauté the onions gently for a few minutes in a small amount of water, stirring regularly to prevent the vegetables sticking.

3. Dissolve the bouillon in the boiling water and pour over the onions. Add the chopped squash and coconut milk and bring to a gentle simmer.

4. Cover and cook for a further 20 minutes until all the vegetables are tender.

5. Blend the soup until smooth, adding more stock if the soup is too thick.

6. Add basil or parsley before serving.

⌐ *Split-pea soup (therapeutic)* ⌐

If you are on a tight budget and you want to add a filling nourishing soup to your menu, this one is both cheap and cheerful. With just three ingredients – peas, onions and vegetable stock – this soup is great value for money. I serve this to friends and family on cold evening or for a satisfying lunch-time filler. It's cheap, easy and delicious.

Serves 4

'Dust with paprika before serving to give the soup a warm and colourful appeal.'

2 cups of dried green split peas

2 onions

1 tablespoon of vegetable bouillon

5 cups of boiling water

Directions

1. Soak the dried peas in cold water for about an hour to soften them. Drain off the soak water.

2. Dissolve the bouillon in the boiling water and pour over the peas. Peel the onions, cut into slices and add to the peas and stock.

3. Bring to a gentle simmer.

4. Cover and cook for a further 20 minutes until all the peas and onions are tender.

5. Blend the soup until smooth, adding more stock if the soup is too thick.

∽ *Chilled carrot and avocado soup (therapeutic)* ∽

This soup is very popular in Cornucopia, Dublin's finest vegetarian restaurant. When they added this raw soup to their menu, people were reluctant to try it – it seemed that a good warming bowl of soup is the traditional cure for winter chills. However, as customers became used to the idea of a chilled carrot soup, news spread and soon this soup was sold out every day. James, the chef, has been more specific about the amounts of ingredients.

Serves 4

'Try substituting with fresh ginger instead of garlic and lemon, you will soon settle on your own personal favourite.'

1 ½ kg carrots (juiced)

1 avocado

4 medium lemons (juiced)

1 clove of peeled garlic

150ml of extra virgin olive oil

Directions

1. Cut the avocado in half and peel and removed the stone.

2. Using a juicer, make the carrot juice.

3. Pour the carrot juice into a blender and add the prepared avocado, and the lemon juice and garlic.

4. Blend to a puree until creamy and well combined.

5. Bring the soup to just under room temperature and then remove from the heat source.

6. Slowly pour in the olive oil and serve.

∽ *Fabulous seaweed soup (therapeutic)* ∽

Seaweeds and avocados are staples among raw-food enthusiasts. This raw seaweed soup is fantastically nutritious and tasty, and, as an added bonus, it's very quick and easy to prepare. It's wonderful if you have an unexpected visitor and have to improvise with store-cupboard ingredients. The coconut and seaweed is a great combination of flavours and the avocado pairs equally well.

Serves 2

'It's such a tasty change from the over-cooked soups that have become the norm in modern-day cooking.'

2 cups of wakame or sea salad

½ a 200-gram block of coconut cream

½ an avocado

1 teaspoon Bragg's Liquid Aminos

½ pint of boiling water

Directions

1. Soak the wakame seaweed in a bowl of tepid water for about 15 minutes while you peel the avocado and chop the block of coconut.
2. Drain the water from the wakame and dry the excess water with a kitchen towel.
3. Blend the wakame, coconut, avocado and Bragg's together.
4. Gradually add boiling water until you get the desired consistency.
5. Serve immediately.

෩ *Mushroom pâté with roasted red pepper salsa (therapeutic)* ෩

Mushrooms are a great addition to vegetarian or vegan dishes as they give a chewy texture which is very satisfying. Some mushrooms are also a rich source of vitamin D, especially shitake. Vitamin D is necessary for absorbing calcium. The courgette strips are rolled into cylinders with the delicious mushroom pâté and topped with the red pepper salsa to add a sweet taste to this yummy pâté.

Serves 1

'Drizzle this salsa over tacos or hummus for that extra sweet flavour.'

12 mushrooms

1 clove of garlic

2 shallots

2 red peppers

2 courgettes

2 tablespoons of olive oil

Directions

1. Slice mushrooms of your choice roughly, add some finely diced garlic, shallots and a little thyme.

2. Place mushroom mix in a pot with a drop of water.

3. Sauté until mushrooms are cooked through.

4. Place in a blender (including the juices). Pulse to a coarse pâté consistency.

5. Roast some red bell peppers in the oven until the skin blisters.

6. Cover peppers in a bowl so that the skin will peel off.

7. Dice the peppers and add a little olive oil to them.

8. Peel strips of courgette with a potato peeler and cook for five seconds in boiling water.

9. Refresh in cold water and pat dry.

10. Place a dollop of mushroom pâté on the courgettes strips and roll into cylinders. Drizzle with the red pepper salsa.

⌒ *Omega rich soup (therapeutic)* ⌒

This is truly a nutritious soup because raw soups retain the enzymes and nutrients that are otherwise lost when they are cooked. If you prefer a warm soup, add some warm water to this recipe. It's the avocado that gives this soup its creamy texture. Avocados are rich in omega-3 fatty acids and vitamin E, which is great for your skin and hair.

Serves 1

'Raw soups are so easy to prepare, you simply throw everything into a blender and whizz. Simple.'

1 avocado

2 small carrots

½ tin of coconut milk

1 teaspoon ginger (finely chopped)

¼ lemon

4–5 drops of stevia (optional)

Pinch of paprika

Directions

1. Peel the avocado, carrots and ginger.

2. Put all the ingredients in a blender and blend until smooth.

3. Add a little warm water if the soup is too thick.

4. Add the paprika just before serving.

⌒ *Beetroot carpaccio with mustard slaw (transition)* ⌒

Beetroot is high in fibre, antioxidants and iron. Soluble fibre has been shown to lower cholesterol and beetroots powerful antioxidants protect the heart. Beetroot is also rich in silica which is good for skin and connective tissues and also bone health. I don't tend to use vinegar as it slows the absorption of nutrients, but this one is great for special occasions. My thanks to Alan at Nautilus restaurant for producing such wonderful food, this is one of my favourite starter at the restaurant.

Serves 2–4

'Don't discard the green leaves of the beetroot, they can be added to juices.'

3 beetroots

2 tablespoon of olive oil

I teaspoon of whole-grain mustard

I tablespoon of white wine vinegar

Handful of chopped dill

I orange (zest)

½ cup of walnuts

Directions

1. Boil the beetroots in their skins until they are tender, allow to cool, peel and slice thinly.

2. Using a pastry or cookie cutter, cut round discs. Chop any trimmings that are left over finely.

3. Put the olive oil, whole-grain mustard, chopped dill, white wine vinegar and orange zest in a bowl and mix well.

4. Toast the walnuts under the grill.

5. Arrange the beetroot discs in a circle in the middle of the plate. Place the beetroot salad in the middle and sprinkle the toasted walnuts on top.

⤝ *Mammy's home-made bread (transition)* ⤜

My mum loved to make fresh bread – the smell of this bread cooking still evokes memories of my mother's kitchen and her delicious baking. She would throw a handful of nutritious seeds into the mix as she loved the crunchy texture it gave to the bread. I am sure she had no idea that flax seeds are high in fibre, or that pumpkin seeds are rich in calcium, B vitamins and essential fatty acids, but she did it anyway.

Makes 1 loaf

'I have been more specific about the amounts as when baking bread, it's important to have the quantities correct.'

340g of brown spelt flour

300ml organic rice milk

1 tablespoon of sesame seeds

3 tablespoons of sunflower seeds

2 tablespoons of pumpkin seeds

3 teaspoons of gluten-free baking powder

½ lemon (juiced)

knob of coconut butter

Directions

1. Preheat the oven to gas mark 4/175°C.

2. Mix all the dry ingredients together, sieving the baking powder into the dry mix.

3. Add the rice milk and lemon juice and mix thoroughly until a thick dough forms.

4. Lightly coat a 450g loaf tin with the coconut butter.

5. Pour the mixture into the tin until it's about three-quarters full.

6. Bake for 45 minutes to an hour.

7. Turn out onto a baking tray and check to see if the base of the loaf is firm.

∽ *Delicious garlic mushrooms (therapeutic)* ∽

I think most people love the taste of garlic mushrooms but they are mostly fried in harmful oils that are not good for your health. Mushrooms are loaded with B vitamins and with the addition of some garlic, you can easily make a healthy starter. I dehydrate these in oil and garlic and voilà, you're done. Wait till you catch the smell of these coming out of the dehydrator.

Serves 2

'The first time I made these, I ate the whole batch myself. They were delicious.'

4 cups of mushrooms

½ cup of extra virgin olive oil

3 garlic cloves

Directions

1. Crush the garlic cloves and add with the oil into a mixing bowl.

2. Clean and slice the mushrooms.

3. Add them to the oil mix and allow the mushrooms to soak up the garlic oil.

4. Dehydrate for 30–40 minutes.

5. Serve with a mixed green salad.

Mains

When you are preparing food, why not make something that will actually nourish your body? Prepare dishes that are good for your health *and* good for your figure.

Remember, ready-made meals are high in sugars and salts. Eating excess sodium can be harmful to people with hypertension or high blood pressure, and it causes fluid retention. Microwave meals may be convenient, but microwaves denature food, so they may fill you and give you calories but the vitamins, minerals and proteins in the food will be destroyed.

I know when you live in a cold climate, the thought of salads and raw foods may not be appealing. Winter weather makes us crave comforting, hot dishes. This is where a dehydrator comes in very handy. It starts the process of eating for health rather than comfort and you can eat warm foods without destroying their valuable nutrients. Here are three tips for eating more raw, living foods throughout the chillier weather:

- add more chilli, cayenne pepper and ginger to your foods.
- warm plates before serving.
- put warm sauces over your salad.

It is so easy to add real, nourishing foods into your day-to-day routine.

1. **Hearty stuffed peppers (therapeutic)**

2. **Roast veggie bake (therapeutic)**

3. **Hot and spicy curry (therapeutic)**

4. **Sautéed Chinese vegetables (therapeutic)**

3. **Nuts about tacos (therapeutic)**

6. **Easy as cottage pie (transition)**

7. **Comforting Irish stew (transition)**

∽ *Hearty stuffed peppers (therapeutic)* ∽

Peppers are great for stuffing, and the stuffing in this recipe is very substantial. If you need some inspiration, this satisfying dish is uncomplicated and truly delicious.

Serves 2

> *'I love the mingling of the herbs with the lemon in this stuffing, it gives this dish that extra smack of flavour.'*

To prepare the peppers:

2 red peppers

¼ cup of tamari sauce

¼ cup of olive oil

Directions

1. Wash and cut the peppers in half and discard the seeds.

2. Marinate in tamari sauce and oil for 20 minutes, turning occasionally.

⌒ *Roast veggie bake (therapeutic)* ⌒

Most people use oil when they roast vegetables to keep them from sticking to the dish they are being cooked in, but as heating fats is not good for our health, I prefer to use water and add the oil after the dish comes off the heat source. You can, of course, eliminate the oil altogether if you prefer, although fats can make food tasty.

Serves 2–4

'This is a sumptuous, heart-warming dish that will light up your inner fire on those cold winter evenings.'

2 red bell peppers

I sweet potato

I butternut squash

I red onion

I tablespoon of fresh thyme

2 tablespoon of fresh rosemary

I tablespoon of vegetable bouillon

¼ cup of water

¼ cup of olive oil

Directions

1. Pre-heat the oven to 180°C.

2. Peel and scoop out the seeds from the squash and peppers and cut into cubes.

3. Peel the remaining veggies and chop them into cubes of about the same size so they will cook evenly.

4. Throw all the veggies onto a baking tray with the chopped herbs.

5. Blend the bouillon with hot water and pour over the vegetables.

6. Bake in the oven until veggies are tender (approximately 40 minutes)

7. Drizzle the oil over the veggies and serve with low-carb rice (see page 218).

To prepare the stuffing:

½ cup of pine nuts

I avocado

½ cup of sweetcorn

I small onion

½ teaspoon of vegetable bouillon

I tablespoon of Udo's oil

Fresh herbs (basil or parsley)

½ lemon (juiced)

Directions

1. In a blender, process the nuts, herbs, avocado, bouillon and onion, adding the oil last.

2. Stuff each pepper evenly with the mixture.

3. Place in dehydrator for I hour 30 minutes.

∽ *Hot and spicy curry (therapeutic)* ∽

In this dish, the yellow lentils are tempered with cumin and chilli to get that authentic curry flavour. The turmeric root is a valued condiment that adds flavour and a pronounced yellow colour to food. Real curry sauces (not from a jar) may appear a little complex at first, but many of the spices they include are ones that you will have in your spice rack. You can always vary this recipe with a different range of seasonal vegetables. Keep sprouted lentils to hand to add to soups, salads and cooked meals, they are great to add extra nutrients and vitamins to the foods you eat.

Serves 2–4

'Sprouting the lentils and adding them just before serving makes this dish more nutritious, alternatively you can use cooked lentils.'

I onion

I butternut squash

I small cauliflower

2 cups of vegetable stock

I cup of yellow lentils (sprouted for two days)

I red chilli

½ teaspoon of ginger

I teaspoon of cumin

¼ teaspoon of turmeric

I teaspoon of curry powder

I tablespoon of gram flour

Directions

1. Put the onion, squash, cauliflower, chilli, ginger, cumin, turmeric and curry powder in a large pot containing, the two cups of vegetable stock.

2. Cook gently for 30 minutes, until the vegetables are soft.

3. Blend the gram flour with a small amount of hot water to make a sauce.

4. Stir in the sprouted lentils just before serving the curry.

⤳ *Sautéed Chinese vegetables (therapeutic)* ⤳

If you are not eating as many veggies as you would like to, try this delicious Chinese meal. It is not fried, so you will get all the benefits of the nutritious ingredients. The addition of bean sprouts and tamari (soy sauce) is reminiscent of Chinese stir frys. Tamari is excellent for quick marinades, you simply add it to some oil. Serve with low-carb rice (see page 218).

Serves 2

'This meal is so easy and quick to prepare. It will soon replace the takeaway.'

1 onion

2 cups of spinach

1 garlic clove

2 cups of bean sprouts

1 cup of mushrooms

1 red pepper

2 tablespoons of tamari

2 tablespoons of olive oil

Directions

1. Chop the mushrooms, onions, garlic and red pepper and place in a large bowl.

2. Add the bean sprouts.

3. Coat the vegetables in tamari and oil and place on a dehydrator tray until the vegetables become warm and slightly softened (approximately half an hour).

❧ *Nuts about tacos (therapeutic)* ❧

These tacos are fun and easy to prepare. They are my absolute favourite – hands down. I tasted these in a raw restaurant in California and devoured the raw tacos along with some scrumptious guacamole. Walnut taco meat may not sound very inviting, but let me tell you, it is delicious. If you are worried that your family will turn up their noses, I guarantee that this taco stuffing will be a hit. I experimented with this recipe on my teenage daughter and she loved them.

Serves 2

> *'Walnuts are rich in omega-3 fatty acids. They also have higher levels of polyphenolic antioxidants than any other edible nut.'*

2 cups of walnuts

1 small onion

1 garlic clove, finely minced

2 tablespoons of fresh parsley

1 teaspoon of Bragg's Liquid Aminos

2 teaspoons of chilli powder

6 large lettuce leaves

Directions

1. Place all the ingredients, except for the lettuce leaves, in a food processor. Blend until finely chopped, but don't over-blend – the nuts should have a crunchy texture.

2. Place the lettuce leaves on a flat surface and add a few spoonfuls of the walnut mixture on top.

3. Pour over some red pepper salsa (see page 198) roll up the leaves and serve.

∽ *Easy as cottage pie (transition)* ∽

This savoury and satisfying pie is chock full of fresh veg and has a tasty, crunchy potato topping. You can use whatever vegetables you like, the ones listed here are suggested to get you started. If you're eating from the therapeutic recipes, you can omit the potatoes.

Serves 2–4

'This hearty meal is destined to become a firm family favourite.'

1 large head of broccoli

1 large onion

6–8 button mushrooms

1 large leek

2 stalks of celery

2–3 large floury potatoes

½ teaspoon of oregano

1 tablespoon of vegetable bouillon

¾ of a litre of water

1 tablespoon of gram flour

2 tablespoons of rice milk

Directions

1. Peel and chop the veggies into bite-size pieces.

2. Sauté the onions in a pot in a small amount of water at a medium heat for about two minutes. Stir continuously to prevent sticking.

3. Blend the vegetable bouillon with the water and pour over the onions.

4. Throw in the veggies and herbs and reduce the heat, allowing the stew to simmer for 30 minutes.

5. Blend the gram flour with a small amount of hot water and add to the vegetables to thicken the sauce.

6. Meanwhile make the mash; first peel and cook the potatoes.

7. Strain the potatoes and mix in the rice milk until the mash is creamy.

8. Place the veggies in a casserole dish and top with the mash.

9. Smooth with a fork and bake under the grill for a few minutes until golden brown.

∽ *Comforting Irish stew (transition)* ∽

This Irish stew can be made with just veggies and is great for using up the leftovers from your fridge. The smell of this delicious stew will make your mouth water. Instead of using bleached white flour to thicken the sauce, I use gram flour, which is made from ground chickpeas and is available in supermarkets and health food stores. The stew can be prepared in advance if you like as it lets the flavours develop. You can also omit the potatoes if you are eating from the therapeutic menus.

Serves 2–4

> *'Even the meat-and-potatoes type will gobble up this scrumptious dish.'*

2 onions

3 carrots

1 leek

1 small turnip

2 tablespoon of vegetable bouillon

¾ of a litre of water

10 new potatoes

1 tablespoon of gram flour

Directions

1. Peel and chop the vegetables into bite-size pieces.
2. Sauté the onions in a pot in a small amount of water for about two minutes. Stir continuously to prevent sticking.
3. Make a stock by blending the vegetable bouillon in the water and then add it to the onions.
4. Throw the veggies, potatoes, stock and herbs into a pot. Bring to the boil and then reduce the heat, allowing the stew to simmer for an hour.
5. Blend the gram flour with a small amount of hot water and then add to the stew to thicken the sauce.

Salads and sides

You don't have to be deprived or live on a leaf of lettuce when you're trying to lose weight. If you want to drop a size, then eating less bread, potatoes and pasta can make a big difference. Reduce the carbs on your plate by adding more veggies to your meals. Switch to my no-calorie spaghetti (see page 219) or my low-carb rice (see page 218), made with veggies, they are filling and taste good. These recipes will help you successfully revolutionise your diet and health permanently. They will also help you embrace eating nourishing food within your busy schedule.

1. **Market green salad (therapeutic)**
2. **Crumbly cheesy topping (therapeutic)**
3. **Tangy beetroot salad (therapeutic)**
4. **Ocean energy salad (therapeutic)**
5. **Low-carb rice (therapeutic)**
6. **No-calorie spaghetti (therapeutic)**
7. **Curry roasted parsnips with a ginger chilli remoulade (therapeutic)**

⌒ *Market green salad (therapeutic)* ⌒

I served this salad with the healthy salad dressing (see page 235) to a large group and they loved it so much, they marked it '11 out of 10' and munched up all the greens. I love the freshness of delicate leaves that are straight from the market onto the table. Even in the dead of winter, when greens are not so abundant, many growers produce salad leaves in glass houses. The mangetout gives a nice crunchy texture to this salad, but you can use sugar-snap peas if you can't get mangetout.

Serves 4

'Crumble some of my cheesy parmesan (see below) over the top of this salad, it's wonderful.'

I large bowl of mixed salad leaves

I cup mangetout

2 cups of sprouted sunflower sprouts

Directions

1. Wash and dry the leaves, sprouts and peas.

2. Combine all the ingredients and drizzle over some healthy salad dressing.

3. Top with crumbly cheesy parmesan.

⤚ *Crumbly cheesy topping (therapeutic)* ⤚

This tastes a bit like parmesan cheese, but is made without any dairy ingredients. The secret ingredient is nutritional yeast, which can be bought in most health stores as well as some supermarkets. Here I have added vegetable bouillon to give the cheese that authentic salty taste. The first time I made this I wasn't quite sure how it would turn out, using yeast was totally new territory for me, but what a yummy surprise.

'You can eat this cheese straight or crumble it over salads and soups. It's truly awesome.'

1 cup of pine nuts

1 cup of macadamia nuts

4 tablespoons of nutritional yeast

½ cup of lemon juice

1 cup of water

1 teaspoon of vegetable bouillon

Directions

1. Soak the nuts in water for half an hour. Drain well and process the nuts in a blender.

2. Add the rest of the ingredients to the blender and process until smooth and creamy.

3. Spread thinly on two sheets of parchment paper or Teflex sheets.

4. Dry overnight in a dehydrator until the cheese is fully dry. Crumble over salads or soups.

∽ *Tangy beetroot salad (therapeutic)* ∽

This is such a lovely addition to any green salad because it has a lovely, tangy flavour. Beetroot is abundant in potassium, magnesium and iron, as well as vitamins C and B6 and folic acid, which is essential to the development of a baby's spinal cord during the first three months of pregnancy. This salad is one of my hubby's favourites.

Serves 2

> *'Beets are loaded with powerful antioxidants and studies show they can reduce blood pressure and the risk of heart attacks and strokes.'*

I fresh beetroot

½ lemon (juiced)

Small piece of ginger

Directions

1. Peel and roughly chop the beetroot and ginger.
2. Add the juice of the lemon and blitz in small chopper for a few seconds and serve.

⌒ *Ocean energy salad (therapeutic)* ⌒

I love the colour of this salad. It has a salty seafood taste and is truly lovely. Here in Ireland, we have a range of high-quality sea vegetables that are harvested from our shores but, despite this, we are reluctant to add them to the weekly menu. Japanese people, on the other hand, make good use of seaweeds with favoured dishes like sautéed hijiki or wakame soup. This neglected vegetable is such a wonderful addition to our diet that it deserves a place on the menu. Put it on your shopping list right now!

Serves 4

'Loaded with minerals, this salad can be mixed together in no time.'

1 200-gram pack of dried dulse seaweed

1 red chilli

10 drops of stevia

3 tablespoons of Udo's oil

1 teaspoon of sprouted sesame seeds

1 teaspoon of Bragg's Liquid Aminos

1 tablespoon of lemon juice

Directions

1. Soak the dulse seaweed in a bowl of tepid water for about 15 minutes while you prepare the other ingredients. The dulse should be totally submerged in the water.

2. Drain off the water and dry the excess water with a towel. Cut the dulse into thin strips and place in a serving dish.

3. Combine the oil, lemon juice, Bragg's and stevia. Pour the dressing over the dulse and toss.

4. Sprinkle with the sprouted sesame seeds and finely chopped chilli.

∽ *Low-carb rice (therapeutic)* ∽

This is great addition to any meal – you can serve it with stir-frys, stir-raw, salads or roast vegetables. It is also delicious served with your favourite curry or with a fresh green salad. Macadamia nuts work well in this recipe as they are quite oily and give a fried rice effect when dehydrated. Rice has very little taste, it's the sauce you add or the food you serve with it that adds flavour. You can add half a teaspoon of curry powder and a handful of raisins to turn this into an attractive pilaf rice.

Serves 2–3

'This rice has been a big hit with my friends and students not only for its taste, but because it is so easy to prepare.'

2 parsnips

¼ cup of macadamia nuts soaked

2 teaspoons of olive oil

Directions

1. Peel the parsnips and place, with the nuts, in a processor and chop finely.

2. Place on parchment paper in a dehydrator until warm (approximately half an hour) and serve.

∽ *No-calorie spaghetti (therapeutic)* ∽

I use a turning slicer to make this no-calorie spaghetti. Invest in one of these inexpensive kitchen gadgets to make interesting curly strands from courgettes, sweet potato, carrots and butternut squash. You will get professional-looking cut vegetables with a simple turn of the handle. Pasta is composed almost entirely of carbohydrates, which can have a huge impact on your waistline. Excess calories make you pile on the pounds.

Serves 1–2

*'The long spirals of sweet potato, carrots or courgettes
will add a nice twist to your salads. No sticky pots to
take care of afterwards.'*

2 courgettes

Directions

1. Trim of the ends of the courgettes and put through the turning slicer with the coarse blade, making a long spiral.

⌐ *Curry-roasted parsnips with a ginger chilli remoulade (therapeutic)* ⌐

There is nothing nicer than a good night out sharing a meal with some friends, and one of my favourite restaurants to eat in my local village is Nautilus. Their chef, Alan, is extremely talented and I really enjoy the different flavours he incorporates into his dishes. I usually ring in advance and he prepares something delicious and healthy for me to enjoy.

Serves 2–4

> *'Parsnips are very economical vegetables. They are also a good source of soluble fibre.'*

6 parsnips

I teaspoon of curry powder

I red chilli

2 tablespoon of olive oil

2 tablespoons of cumin seeds

Small piece of ginger

Bunch of coriander

Directions

1. Pre-heat the oven to 180°C.

2. Peel the parsnips, then cut one third off the thin end and reserve for the remoulade. Cut that large ends lengthways in half, sprinkle with curry powder and bake until tender.

3. Take the parsnips off the heat source and drizzle with a little olive oil.

For the remoulade:

1. Grate the thin end of the parsnip, and add grated ginger, finely diced red chilli (no seeds) and chopped coriander.

2. In a dry pan, toast the cumin seeds until they start to pop. Add them to the raw parsnip then add a little olive oil and whole grain mustard to bind.

3. Arrange the warm-roasted parsnips on a plate going head to toe. Place spoonfuls of remoulade on top.

Crisps and crackers

They're fried in fat and covered in salt, but still we eat an enormous 5 billion packets of them a year. *Heart-clogging* as this may be, its pretty obvious that we have an unhealthy addiction to crisps of all kinds. Cheese and onion, salt and vinegar, spicy tortilla, prawn cocktail, barbecue, sweet chilli, char-grilled chicken, balsamic vinegar – there are so many flavours to choose from. We put them in sandwiches, eat them straight from the bag and once we start, we can't stop.

Crisps that are fried and heated in oils have a terrible impact on our health. Heating oils at high temperatures changes their structure into twisted molecules called trans-fatty acids. Fried fats cause a hardening of the arteries and makes blood platelets sticky. They increase the danger of free-radical damage and may cause pathogenic problems.

If the idea of making your own crisps doesn't spark your fire, that may be because you assume that making them is difficult. Let me tell you it's *not*. With a small investment in a dehydrator, an inexpensive drying machine (see the resources section, page 244), you can make crisps, snacks, biscuits, crackers and main meals that will produce satisfying, tasty and enzyme-rich foods for yourself and your family. It's worth the investment just for the crisps alone.

Don't be put off by the length of time it takes to dry the foods. The time is not spent preparing the food, it's just the length of time it takes to dry out the foods. A dehydrator is not like an oven, there is no risk of burning the food in one so you don't have to watch over it.

The following are super-healthy snacks for you to enjoy if you get the munchies while watching TV or sitting at your desk, and they are great for kid's lunchboxes. You can buy some of these crisps in speciality stores, but it is much more economical to make you own.

1. **Salty parsnip crisps (therapeutic)**

2. **Sweet potato crisps (therapeutic)**

3. **Something to chew on (therapeutic)**

4. **Bags of tasty onion rings (therapeutic)**

5. **Scrumptious spinach crisps (therapeutic)**

6. **Fire crackers (therapeutic)**

7. **Tasty apple crisps (transition)**

8. **Lovely onion crackers (therapeutic)**

ᔟ *Salty parsnip crisps (therapeutic)* ᔟ

If you are a crisp addict, this is a wonderful alternative to fried potato crisps. I use salted vegan bouillon for this recipe which gives the crisps an authentic flavour. You can use a reduced salt bouillon if you prefer. The purchase of an inexpensive dehydrator is worth it for these crisps alone. They are delicious served with Julie's yummus or no-cheese basil pesto (see page 233).

'I don't use the centre of the parsnip as it is too tough for crisps. I make the no-carb rice from the leftovers.'

2 parsnips

I tablespoon of vegetable bouillon

¾ cup of hot water

Directions

1. Mix the bouillon and water.

2. Slice the parsnips thinly and dip in boullion mix.

3. Place on dehydrator tray.

4. Dry until crisp turning once during the drying process.

∽ *Sweet potato crisps (therapeutic)* ∽

These crisps are a great snack to have on hand when hunger strikes. Sweet potato crisps are delicious served with some pesto, hummus or tapenade. They have a low glycaemic load, are rich in vitamin A, and also provide fibre and vitamin C. I find that the minute they are prepared, they disappear quickly, especially when my son Richard is around.

'This is a scrummy snack that you won't feel guilty about scoffing.'

2 sweet potatoes

3 tablespoons of salted vegetable bouillon

1 cup of hot water

Directions

1. Wash and slice the sweet potatoes thinly, with the skins on.
2. Blend the vegetable bouillon with the hot water.
3. Coat the sliced sweet potatoes in the bouillon.
4. Place on dehydrator until crisp.

∽ *Something to chew on (therapeutic)* ∽

Kale is one of most the nutrition vegetables there is. It's versatile in side dishes, main dishes or in salads, but it's absolutely fabulous for crisps. Kale is also an excellent source of nutrients, especially vitamin A, beta-carotene and calcium. It's a great immune booster that provides important nutrients for those battling against cancer, heart disease and certain age-related, chronic diseases. Kale is high in fibre which helps create the bulk you need to fill you up.

'If you want to lose weight but still yearn for the salty taste of crisps, this recipe is perfect for you.'

1 bunch of kale

1 tablespoon of vegetable bouillon

½ cup of olive oil

Directions

1. Remove the kale from its stalks.

2. Combine the oil and the veggie bullion. Lightly coat the kale in the mixture and place on dehydrator tray.

3. Dry until crisp, turning once during the drying process.

∽ *Bags of tasty onion rings (therapeutic)* ∽

The kids in school swapped chocolate with my daughter Julie for these onion rings, which really let me know I had got this recipe just right. The simple combination of onions and sweetcorn is fantastic. These are an ideal complement for dips on a night in front of the telly.

'If you're looking for bags of taste from your crisps, these onion rings are the perfect solution.'

3 white onions

2 cups frozen sweetcorn

1 tablespoon of salted vegetable bouillon

¼ cup of water

Directions

1. Blend the sweetcorn and vegetable bouillon together until it forms a creamy batter.

2. Add some water to the batter if it is too thick, though you do need a fairly thick consistency.

3. Slice the onions into fairly thick rings and coat the onions rings in the batter.

4. Place the coated onions rings on a dehydrator tray and dry till crisp, turning once.

⤚ *Scrumptious spinach crisps (therapeutic)* ⤚

These are great to have at hand for emergencies if you get a craving or are particularly partial to the saltiness of potato crisps. If you are constantly grazing and snacking but you want something healthy, these will rival your favourite fried crisps.

'They are so yummy you may not want to share.'

1 120-gram bag of baby spinach leaves

2 cups of sweetcorn

1 onion

1 tablespoon of salted vegetable bouillon

¼ cup of water

Directions

1. Blend the sweetcorn, onion and vegetable bouillon together until you have a creamy batter.

2. Add some water to the batter if it is too thick, though you do need a fairly thick consistency.

3. Coat just one side of the spinach leaves with the batter. Don't coat both sides as they will stick to the tray.

4. Place in a dehydrator tray, with the sticky side up to avoid sticking. Dry till crisp.

∽ *Fire crackers (therapeutic)* ∽

I am not into long lists of ingredients and this recipe has such a long list that it may seem like it's not worth the hassle when crackers are so readily available in the stores. Firstly, most crackers have hidden sugars and hydrogenated fats in them and, second these ingredients are nutritious – you know exactly what in the crackers you're eating. And last but not least, you cannot compare the delicious taste of home-made crackers with the store-bought varieties.

Makes about 24

'I use some of the dried buckwheat that I make for breakfast to add a crunchy texture to the crackers.'

2 cups of buckwheat (sprouted and dehydrated)

2 cups of buckwheat (sprouted but *not* dried)

2 red peppers

2 onions

4 sticks of celery

2 leeks

3 cloves of garlic

I large lemon (juiced)

I teaspoon of cayenne pepper

3 teaspoons of oregano

3 tablespoons of vegetable bouillon

3 tablespoons of psyllium husk

2 level teaspoons of cumin

Directions

1. Blend all the ingredients, except the dried buckwheat.

2. Add a little water to combine into a dough-like consistency.

3. Adjust the flavouring to suit your taste, and then add the dried buckwheat. Be careful with the cayenne pepper if you don't like hot spicy foods.

4. Spread onto parchment paper and score square shapes into the dough. This makes it easy to break the crackers when they are dry.

5. Dehydrate overnight until dry and crispy.

⇆ *Tasty apple crisps (transition)* ⇆

Just slice the apples, dip them in lemon juice to stop discoloration and pop them in a dehydrator. Get the kids to pitch in with a helping hand making these crisps – remember kids always feel so proud of what they have made themselves. Drying concentrates the apple's sweetness, so experiment with different varieties of apple. They are great for kid's lunchboxes.

'These sweet crispy slices are tinged with just the slightest bit of tartness from the lemon, a delicious combination.'

3 apples

1 lemon (juiced)

Directions

1. You can use a mandoline to slice the apples, but mind your fingers. Alternatively just use a sharp knife.

2. Core the apples but don't waste the seeds, they can be add to your juice as they contain nitrosilide compounds that protect us against disease.

3. Dip the apple slices in the lemon juice and place the slices on the dehydrator.

4. Dry until they have a consistency somewhere between chewy and crunchy.

↝ *Lovely onion crackers (therapeutic)* ↜

These crackers have a chewy texture and work really well with hummus and dips. You can also spread them with avocado or tapenade or simply eat them with your favourite salad. Vary the recipe by adding celery or carrot if you feel the onion is too strong for your taste. These crackers are lovely!

Makes 18 crackers

> *'Chia seeds are an amazing source of omega-3 fatty acids, they are also rich in fibre and proteins.'*

2 white onions

1 garlic clove

2 cups of chia seeds

1 cup of ground sunflower seeds

¼ cup of Bragg's Liquid Aminos

¼ cup of olive oil

½ red chilli finely chopped

2 cups of water

Directions

1. Soaked the sunflower and chia seeds separately in two cups of water overnight.

2. Rinse off the sunflower seeds but use all the gelatinous chia seeds mix.

3. Peel the onions and chop them finely in a processer.

4. Mix the onions with the remaining ingredients until completely combined.

5. Spread the mixture thinly over two sheets of parchment.

6. Score into the mixture with a pizza cutter into square or horizontal shapes.

7. Dehydrate overnight, if the crackers are not fully dry return them to dehydrator until drying is complete.

Dips and dressings

Many salad dressings are laced with large amounts of high-fructose corn syrup, a sugar derivative, and this can increase LDL cholesterol (bad cholesterol), which is a risk factor for cardiovascular disease. Remember the more sugars that are added to your food, the more of it you are consuming.

Try these uncomplicated and delicious recipes. Some of these recipes you can make in minutes, which is great if you have a busy lifestyle and have little time for preparation. I hope they will bring sustainable changes to your life that you will want to stick with and continue your progression towards a healthy lifestyle.

1. **Julie's yummus (therapeutic)**
2. **No-cheese basil pesto (therapeutic)**
3. **Black olive tapenade (therapeutic)**
4. **Healthy salad dressing (therapeutic)**
5. **Cool guacamole sauce (therapeutic)**

∽ *Julie's yummus (therapeutic)* ∽

Hummus is a popular Middle Eastern dip and this recipe is a constant favourite with my daughter, Julie – though we played around with it until we got it just right. If you like spicy food, you can add some finely chopped red chilli to add a bit of colour and swirl a drizzle of olive oil over it just before serving. It keeps for three days if the fridge. You can make it with sprouted chick peas if you want to make a raw hummus.

Serves 4

'Served with a selection of vegetable crudités, hummus makes a great snack or appetiser.'

I garlic clove (crushed)

I 240-gram can chickpeas (drained)

2 tablespoons of tahini (sesame seed paste)

½ lemon (juiced)

2 tablespoon of extra virgin olive oil

I teaspoon of fresh coriander (chopped)

Pinch of cayenne pepper

Directions

1. Place all the ingredients in a food processor, but reserve a few chickpeas for serving.

2. Blend into a smooth mix.

3. Season to taste with a pinch of cayenne pepper and serve topping with reserved chickpeas.

✑ *No-cheese basil pesto (therapeutic)* ✑

This pesto works great over pasta and salads or on crackers. Parmesan cheese is usually one of the main ingredients in pesto, but, as the name suggests, this recipe has no cheese. I use a teaspoon of nutritional yeast to give the pesto that cheesy taste. You can use walnuts or sunflower seeds instead of pine nuts as, pine nuts can be expensive. To be honest, it's difficult to tell the difference in taste.

Serves 1

'The magic of this recipe is the fresh basil. It smells delicious and so will the pesto. Try it you will love it.'

I bunch of fresh basil

I cup of pine nuts

I clove of garlic

1–2 tablespoons of extra virgin olive oil

½ a lemon (juiced)

I teaspoon of nutritional yeast

Directions

1. Process all the ingredients, except the olive oil.

2. Gradually drizzle in the olive oil until the pesto turns to a rough paste.

⤳ *Black olive tapenade (therapeutic)* ⤳

I like to spread tapenade over veggie crackers for a quick snack. Tapenade also makes a great appetiser, and is delicious as a salad topping or served as hors d'oeuvres at a party. You can vary the recipe by using some green olives or some freshly chopped herbs. Olives are high in sodium but they are also a good source of healthy fats.

Serves 1

'Tapenade keeps well when refrigerated, that is if there are any leftovers.'

1 cup of black olives

2 cloves of garlic

2 tablespoons of olive oil

1 teaspoon of lemon juice

Directions

1. Process all ingredients into a rough paste before gradually adding the olive oil.

✐ *Healthy salad dressing (therapeutic)* ✐

A good dressing can make a huge difference to a salad. My dear friend Geraldine shared this recipe for her favourite healthy dressing. You can half the recipe if you like to make your dressing fresh, although this one will keep nicely for three days in the fridge.

Serves 4

> *'Go easy on the cayenne pepper, as it can overpower the dressing.'*

4 tablespoons of Udo's oil

4 tablespoons of olive oil

2 tablespoons of Bragg's Liquid Aminos

2 tablespoons of chopped onion

¼ teaspoon of cayenne pepper

2 cloves of garlic

I lemon (juiced)

A few sprigs of fresh parsley (or any fresh herb)

Directions

1. Whizz the lot in a blender.

2. Adjust flavourings to suit your taste and pour over your favourite salad.

∽ *Cool guacamole sauce (therapeutic)* ∽

I serve this guacamole with nuts about tacos (see page 209) as it cools down the fiery taste of the spicy tacos. I add some extra oil so that the guacamole spoons easily over the tacos. Keep in mind that avocados discolour quickly, so make the guacamole just before serving.

Serves 4

'Avocados are a good source of essential fats they are also rich in beta-carotene and vitamins C and E.'

2 ripe avocados

1 clove of garlic

1 small onion

1 lemon (juiced)

3 teaspoon of olive oil

Directions

1. Peel the avocado and remove the stone.

2. Place the avocado flesh in a small processor with the garlic clove, onion and lemon juice.

3. Blend in the oil until smooth and has a saucy consistency and serve immediately.

Treats

Sugar and chocolate are synonymous with pleasure, but why not make them with something nutritious like nuts and dried fruits?

The idea of going without a treat is not easy. Such is sugar's sweet temptation that we ignore the devastating affect it has on our health. There are many artificial sweeteners which people use as alternatives to sugar but not only are some of these toxic, some of them can actually stimulate your appetite and increase your cravings for sugar – which is all bad news for your health and your waistline.

None of these recipes apply to people eating for therapeutic reasons because even though they are made with natural sugars, they are still recognised as sugar in the body. However, depending on the severity of your condition an occasional treat could be tolerated.

If you transitioning and are trying to overcome a tendency to have too many sugary treats, a weekend treat can train your mind to adjust and help you become less dependent on your sugar fix. The secret is to make it a treat – not a habit.

1. **Guilty pleasures (transition)**

2. **Spoil yourself cookies (transition)**

3. **Heavenly macaroons (transition)**

4. **Just a little sorbet treat (transition)**

5. **Tempting almond torte (transition)**

6. **Sweet date syrup (transition)**

∽ *Guilty pleasures (transition)* ∽

When you begin to balance your blood sugars, you will start thinking logically and rationally about your treats. Mind you, you may not be so rational when you taste these guilty pleasures. I coat them in coconut for extra flavour. The skin of citrus fruit is actually the most beneficial part as it contains the most vitamin C and bioflavonoids.

'Remember these melt-in-the-mouth pleasures may be seductive but keep them for a treat or they may soon become your guilty pleasure.'

2 cups of almonds (soaked and rinsed)

1 cup of sultanas (soaked in orange juice)

½ cup of desiccated coconut

Juice and rind of 1 orange

Directions

1. Blend all ingredients (except the desiccated coconut) through the blank screen provided with your juicer or use a blender.

2. Roll out into balls and coat each ball in desiccated coconut.

3. Refrigerate for 1 hour and try to share!

∽ *Spoil yourself cookies (transition)* ∽

These cookies are so yummy you may want to keep them all for yourself. Save them for those moments when you need an extra bit of TLC. This is probably the easiest recipe for cookies around, they are so simple – you just simply mix the ingredients together. The lemon rind gives them a real zing. These cookies are organic, vegan, dairy and gluten free. Don't be put off by the length of time they take to dry, they really are scrumptious.

Makes 24 cookies

> *'You can dehydrate these cookies overnight if you prefer a crunchier cookie.'*

4 cups pecans nuts (soaked overnight)

I cup of dates (soaked in the juice of a lemon)

5 tablespoons of almond nut butter

Rind of a lemon

Directions

1. Soak the nuts overnight in water and drain. Also soak the dates overnight in the juice of the lemon. Save the rind. The dates will absorb most of the juice.

2. Chop the rind in your processer, then add the nuts, dates and almond butter. Add more almond butter if necessary to bring the mixture together.

3. Form into cookie shapes and place in the dehydrator for three hours. Enjoy!

❦ *Heavenly macaroons (transition)* ❦

These are a mega favourite with my two girls and there is always a scramble for the last one. Various cultures around the world revere the coconut as a valuable source of both food and medicine. It can be used to treat a wide variety of health problems, such as bruises, burns, colds, gingivitis, nausea and sore throats. You can buy the coconut cream in packs in most health stores. The recipe for date syrup is on page 243.

Makes 24 macaroons

'These macaroons are easy to prepare in advance and the carob will hopefully satisfy choccie cravings.'

2 200-gram packs of coconut cream

1 cup carob powder

1 cup date syrup

½ cup coconut butter

1 tablespoon of natural vanilla essence

Directions

1. Mix all the ingredients together until they are well combined and refrigerate for half an hour.

2. Scoop into small balls and place on dehydrator.

3. Dry overnight in the dehydrator until the macaroons are crisp to touch on the outside and soft in the centre.

∽ *Just a little sorbet treat (transition)* ∽

With no colourings or no artificial flavourings, this scrumptious sorbet is a perfect treat. Red grapes are rich in polyphenols, a compound found in foods that are purple or red in colour and which protects your body from cell damage. They are also found in strawberries, raspberries and cranberries. If you own an ice-cream maker you can easily whizz this together.

Serves 4

'This sorbet is a perfect antidote for the sugar blues.'

4 cups of red grapes

10 drops of stevia

½ cup of pure water

Directions

1. Blend all the ingredients in a blender until smooth.

2. Sieve through a fine mesh strainer to eliminate any pulp.

3. Chill for two hours and serve.

❦ *Tempting almond torte (transition)* ❦

Rich and decadent, this two-layer torte tastes very like Christmas pudding and is ideal for special occasions, such as birthdays or Christmas. It's gluten-free and a good source of healthy proteins. I use my masticating juicer for this torte as it binds the ingredients together nicely, but you could use a blender.

Serves 6

> *'You simply cannot go wrong it with this torte it comes out perfect every time.'*

Directions

For the frosting:

I cup dates (pitted)

I lemon

1. Soak the pitted dates in the juice of the lemon, and retain the rind. Let the dates soak up the juice for about one hour, or overnight if you prefer.

2. Chop the rind finely and mix the dates and rind together in a blender.

For the filling:

4 cups of almonds

3 cups of raisins

I lemon

Water to soak

1. Soak the almonds in water overnight. Drain and discard the soak water.

2. Soak the raisins separately in lemon juice and retain the rind.

3. Chop the rind finely and alternate the almonds, raisins and lemon rind through the juicer or blend together.

4. Press half the mixture into an eight- or nine-inch spring-form tin.

5. Layer over a third of the frosting and add the remaining filling.

6. Chill for half an hour and press the torte out onto a serving plate.

7. Coat the outside of the torte with the remaining frosting and serve.

⌒ *Sweet date syrup (transition)* ⌒

Dates are natural sweeteners, but they are still recognised as sugars by your body and should still be eaten in moderation. I prefer Medjool dates, but this can be made successfully with the smaller varieties. Lemon juice adds a nice tangy flavour and helps to keep the syrup fresh (it will keep for two weeks when refrigerated).

'I like to add some vanilla extract or some cinnamon
for extra flavour.'

2 cups of Medjool dates (pitted)

1 tablespoon of lemon juice

Grated cinnamon or vanilla essence to taste

Directions

1. Blend the ingredients through your juicer or use a blender until you have a smooth consistency.

Resources

You can contact Bernadette on:
telephone: (00 353) (0)1-845-2957
email: b@changesimply.com
website: www.changesimply.com
www.facebook/changesimply
www.twitter.com/bernadettebohan
www.linkedin.com/bernadettebohan

Hippocrates Health Institute
telephone: 00-1-516-471-8876
website: www.hippocrates.inst.com
address: 1443 Palmdale Court, West Palm Beach, Florida, 33411, USA

Reverse osmosis systems by Renewell Water Group
telephone: (00 353) (0)86-733-5874
email: info@renewellwater.com
website: www.renewellwater.com

Wheatgrass and fresh sprouts delivery services
Christy Stapleton
telephone: (00 353) (0)59-647-3460 or (00 353) (0)86-103-8605
email: christystap@gmail.com
website: www.christysorganicwheatgrass.ie

The Happy Pear Living Foods
telephone: (00 353) (0)86-101-4181
email: sprouts@livingfoods.ie
website: www.livingfoods.ie

Quickcrop.ie Organic Growers
telephone: (00 353) (0)1-524-0084 (for Ireland) and
(00 44) (0)178-829-8795 (for the UK)

Thermal imaging

Liz Nagle ND
telephone: (00 353) (0)86-811-4073
website: www.onehealth.ie

Safe personal care products

Naturamatics
telephone: (00 353) (0)86-199-9842
email: info@naturamatics.com
website: www.naturamatics.com

Other useful websites

www.irelandagainstfluroidation.org
http://homepage.eircom.net/~fluoridefree/20reasons.htm
www.cornucopia.ie (vegetarian restaurant in Dublin)

Improve your health naturally

Three-day residential wellness programme

Since I began my wellness programme, thousands of people have come to learn the practical, powerful and effective healing steps of my course. It is designed to cultivate a healthy lifestyle in a unique and permanent way. It is ideal for people who are facing health issues or for those who wish to simply improve their health. The results have been very encouraging and the positive feedback highlights that many guests have experienced their tumour markers tumbling downwards, have less reliance on painkillers and have a general feeling of health with increased energy levels.

Using a nutritional approach, the programme introduces a way of living that leads to sustainable good health. The combination of a nutritional diet of organic foods, health education classes, food demonstrations of delicious, healthy meals and meditation, enables a deep experience of wellbeing. Increased energy levels and glowing skin are just small pieces of the jigsaw that you will experience.

On my residential programme, the tranquil atmosphere provides not only the ideal location to totally unwind but also the ideal environment to focus on improving your health. So if you feel you're not quite firing on all cylinders, join me and recharge our batteries. You will leave rejuvenated and refreshed and grateful you took those three days to take care of yourself.

Non-residential Dublin programme

In response to the ever-growing need for a Dublin-based programme, I have set up a non-residential course where you can learn the various essential steps which are the essence of my programme. These simple steps will transform your life for the better. This is not a diet, it's a way of life, and it will help you improve your food choices, break harmful habits and create better ones. True health must be earned, there are no magic pills or cures that can replace the wonderful foods that nature has given to us. If you have made repeated resolutions to get healthy but have lacked the motivation, willpower and knowledge, then let's get you back on track.

I want to pass on the common-sense steps that helped me return to good health. The process of eating healthily doesn't have to be complicated. In fact, as I have said repeatedly, the secret is to keep it simple – that way you are far more likely to succeed. This lifestyle is sustainable and uncomplicated; believe me if I can do it, so can you. I hope it will become the foundation of informed decision-making and will help you to take responsibility for your health. I hope to see you soon.

For bookings, call (00 353) (0)1-845-2957

Join my newsletter at www.changesimply.com for more juicing recipes, updates and great tips to keep you on track. It will encourage and motivate you, so stay in touch.

Bibliography and further reading

Bibliography

Belcaro G., Cesarone M. R., Dugall M., Pellegrini L., Ledda A., Grossi, M. G., Togni, S. and Appendino, G. (2010). 'Product-evaluation registry of Meriva®, curcumin-phosphatidylcholine complex, for the complementary management of osteoarthritis'. *PanMinerva Med.* 52, suppl. 1 to no. 1, 55–62.

Campbell, Dr Colin T. and Campbell, C. (2005). *The China Study.* Dallas, TX: BenBella Books.

Cho, E., Curhan, G., Hankinson, S. E., Kantoff, P., Atkins, M. B., Stampfer, M. and Choueiri, T. K. (2011). 'Prospective Evaluation of Analgesic Use and Risk of Renal Cell Cancer'. *Archives of Internal Medicine,* 171 (16), 1487–1493.

Drinking Water Inspectorate (2011). 'Review of the risks posed to drinking water by man-made nanoparticles'. York: Food and Environment Research Agency.

Esselstyn, Dr Caldwell (2007). *Prevent and Reverse Heart Disease.* New York: Penguin Group.

Jethro Kloss, J. (2004). *Back to Eden (second edition).* Twin Lakes, WI: Lotuspress.

Kauffman, Joel M. (2005). 'Water Fluoridation: a Review of Recent Research and Actions'. *Journal of American Physicians and Surgeons*, vol. 10, no. 2, 38–44.

Kerrigan, A. M. and Kingdon, C. (2010), 'Maternal obesity and pregnancy: a retrospective study'. *Midwifery*, vol. 26, no. 1, 138–146.

National Health Service (2010). 'Statistics on obesity, physical activity and diet: England'. Leeds: The Health and Social Care Information Centre.

Ornish, Dr Dean (1997). *Love and Survival.* New York: HarperCollins Publisher.

Pert, Dr Candace (1997). *Molecules of Emotion.* New York: Scribner.

Royal College of Physicians (2013). 'Action on obesity: comprehensive care for all', report of a working party. London: RCP.

World Cancer Research Fund (2001). *Food, Nutrition, Physical Activity, and the Prevention of Cancer: a Global Perspective.* London: World Cancer Research Fund.

Yang B., Wang J., Tang B., Liu Y., Guo C., et al. (2011). 'Characterization of Bioactive Recombinant Human Lysozyme Expressed in Milk of Cloned Transgenic Cattle'. *PLoS ONE*, 6(3): e17593. doi:10.1371/journal.pone.0017593.

Further reading

Antczak, Dr S. and Antczak, G. (2001). *Cosmetics Unmasked.* New York, NY: Thorsons.

Barnard, Dr Neal D. (2008). *The Cancer Survivor's Guide.* Summertown, TN: Book Publishing Company.

Bernay-Roman, A. (2001). *Deep Feeling, Deep Healing.* Jupiter, FL: Spectrum Healing Press.

Binzel, E. (1994). *Alive and Well.* Baton Rouge, FL: American Media.

Brazier, B. (2004). *Thrive.* Providence, RI: Oceanside.

Burney, L. (2004). *Immunity Foods for Healthy Kids.* London: Duncan Baird Publishers.

Caldara, L. (2006). *180 Ways to Effectively Deal With Change.* Flower Mound, TX: Walk The Talk Company.

Clement, Dr A.-M. and Clement, Dr B. (2011). *Killer Clothes.* Las Vegas, NV: Hippocrates Publishing Company.

Clement, B. (1998). *Living Foods for Optimum Health.* Rocklin, CA: Prima Health.

Daniel, Dr R. (2003). *Eat to Beat Cancer.* New York, NY: Thorsons.

Daniel, Dr R. (2005). *The Cancer Directory.* New York, NY: Thorsons.

Day, P. (1999). *Cancer: Why we're still Dying to Know the Truth.* London: Credence.

d'Raye, T. (1995). *What's the Big Deal About Water?* Keizer, OR: The Ten Minute Read Company.

Edgson, V. and Marber, I. (1999). *The Food Doctor.* London: Collins & Brown.

Erasmus, U. (1993). *Fats that Heal, Fats that Kill.* Burnaby, BC: Alive Books.

Groves, B. (2001). *Fluoride Drinking Ourselves to Death.* Dublin: Gill & Macmillan.

Gursche, S. (1997). *Encyclopaedia of Natural Healing.* Burnaby, BC: Alive Books.

Gursche, S. (2000). *Juicing – For the Health of It.* Burnaby, BC: Alive Books.

Holford, P. (2007). *Optimum Nutrition for the Mind.* London: Piatkus.

Kahuna Kupua A'o, L. (1996). *Don't Drink the Water.* Pagosa Springs, CO: Kali Press.

Leggett, D. (1999). *Recipes for Self-Healing.* New York, NY: Meridian Press.

McEoin, B. (2001). *Boost Your Immune System Naturally.* London: Carlton.

Melcombe, L. (2000). *Health Hazards of White Sugar.* Burnaby, BC: Alive Books.

Mercola, Dr J. (2004). *Total Health.* www.mercola.com.

O'Bannon, K. (2000). *Sprouts.* Burnaby, BC: Alive Books.

Ornish, Dr. D. (1996). *Programme for Reversing Heart Disease.* New York, NY: Ivy Books.

Plant, J. (2000). *Your Life in Your Hands.* London: Virgin.

Plant, J. A. and Tidey, G. (2001). *The Plant Programme.* London: Virgin.

Simonton, C. (1992). *Getting Well Again.* New York, NY: Bantam.

Steinman, D. and Epstein, S. (1995). *The Shoppers' Bible.* San Francisco, CA: Wiley Publishing Inc.

Taubert, P. M. (2001). *Silent Killers – more than you paid for*. Murray Bridge, South Australia: CompSafe Consultancy.

Thomas, P. (2001). *Cleaning Yourself to Death*. Dublin: Gill & McMillan.

Vale, J. (2002). *Slim 4 Life*. New York, NY: Thorsons.

Vale, J. (2003). *The Juice Master's Ultimate Fast Food*. New York, NY: Thorsons Element.

Vale, J. (2004). *Chocolate Busters*. New York, NY: Thorsons.

Walker, Dr N. (1995). *Water Can Undermine Your Health*. Prescott, AR: Norwalk Press.

Weil, A. (1995). *Spontaneous Healing*. London: Little Brown.

Wheater, C. (2001). *Juicing for Health*. New York, NY: Thorsons.

Index